RN

by

Katie MacInnis, RN

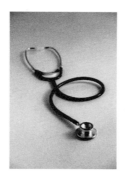

Published in the United States by
Kathleen G. MacInnis
Harbor Springs, Michigan

ISBN 0-9778171-0-5

First Edition

FOREWORD

This little book has a lot of sad stories and ones of complaint. As I put it together, it seemed to need balance, humor, romance, some gimmick to distract the reader so they wouldn't put it down in disgust. But then I thought: you're a grownup, you don't need a note from your mother and, anyway, hadn't you thought about upping your dose of Prozac?

The stories are either about the morgue or complain about what most people do before getting there: retire. I love nursing, and find it hard to consider leaving, but I know I will soon have to hang it up.

Every time I go to work, I am amazed that I am allowed to be someone's nurse, to be there when things happen. I hope this comes through in my stories: that this is an incredible profession, a great choice if you want to work very hard and to know you make a difference. All of these people are real. I didn't make them up. And my stories are like any other nurse's, except that I had the presence of mind to write them down.

We need new nurses. Young people disillusioned with their lives, looking for something that says, each day, they really helped someone. In the years I was published by nursing journals, the only stories they turned away were the ones I wrote criticizing the hyperbole of hospitals trying to attract nurses to their doors. "Come to XYZ

Hospital to be a STAR!" Not one advertisement ever said, "Come and help orient the confused, walk the elderly to the bathroom and wipe bottoms..." But often, it was doing those things that made me feel the best. Something about doing a real thing that really needed doing to help a fellow human.

All too soon, young nurses will be assigned to my room, somewhere. These fledgling nurses will remind me who I am, where I am, and give me my morning pills crushed in applesauce. I hope these nurses are gentle and kind.

Sometimes all I can see in my peripheral vision is death and disease, loss and life changes that speak of endings. This little book lets down the side rails of the bed, and tells the stories that fall out. I cannot be responsible for what happened in the stories, but it feels somehow wrong not tell them. Most of these people would have no memorial or remembrance if not for the words on these pages.

HUMAN DIFFERENCES

Many years ago, as a student nurse doing an obstetrics/pediatric rotation, I was assigned to a mother-child pair. This family was from another country and barely spoke our language.

All had gone well: the baby was content, the mother was doing fine. I was sure they were the picture-perfect OB story, a relief for me in my student days. But by the second day, a stream of visitors began arriving. Uncles, cousins and an assortment of brothers-in-law, all male. Each one took great pleasure in congratulating the mother and father on the birth of their son. Then, at one point during the visit, the parents would carefully release the child's diaper so that each guest could either admire or pat the baby's genitals. Once done, they nodded and bowed to each other and took their leave.

And so my education in human differences began. I was learning to help others, even when I did not personally understand.

Later, when I worked med/surg, a 40-year-old woman named Leslie was near death after a long battle with cancer. All the members of her large family belonged to a charismatic group that believed in miracle healings. They frequently repeated from memory the entire Bible story of Lazarus being raised from the dead.

The nurse taking care of Leslie knew this family would need a lot of time for prayer and meditation to work through their feelings. But when Leslie actually died, there were more than a hundred people who wanted to pray together at her bedside. It was their belief that the united prayer of so many would heal Leslie then and there. Even after the doctor pronounced her dead, they would not discuss post-mortem plans.

A very kind supervisor made arrangements for them. The nurse was freed up from her regular patient assignment. Leslie was transported to the auditorium and her family gathered around the bed to continue their litany. A piano which happened to be close by was used to accompany the many hymns they sang. After about an hour, the family gradually gave up. They seemed to be at peace, although some still thought she would rise up in a few days' time. They thanked us over and over and then, finally, gave us the name of a funeral home.

I was proud to work for that hospital. Even if I could not subscribe to the beliefs of this family, I knew we had done the right thing.

Recently in the ICU, I had to help a young woman deal with sudden death. Steven was 47 to the day when he grabbed his chest and called out to his girlfriend, "Something's wrong, Lisa!" She took him to the ED of an outlying hospital and, though they tried to stabilize him there, his vital signs began to deteriorate. When he arrived at our hospital, he was ashen, clammy and had a systolic blood pressure of 60. This was Steven's big one. We took him to the cath lab and there, what little heart muscle he had, quivered to a standstill. No matter that we gave him drugs, CPR, the balloon pump. He was gone.

I was the first one to see Lisa as we walked passed the waiting room afterward. She had heard the code paged overhead. When she saw my face, she began to wail: "He died? He died! Oh no!" All I could tell her was, "Yes, I'm so very sorry."

"I want to see him," she begged. "Of course," I told her. For long moments we waited for the cath lab personnel to bring him up to the ICU room. Then Lisa began her goodbyes. She gently laid her head on his chest and cried: "I love you so, I love you so."

I asked if she would like to be alone. She said yes, but asked if she could see him one last time. "I mean, can I look at all of him?" It took me a minute, but when she added, "He was so beautiful; we had a good thing together," I thought I understood. "Of course, Lisa, take all the time you need."

It felt like I had done this before, years ago, in my student days.

She was with him for about five minutes. When she left his room, she seemed to be in control. A few weeks later, I got a letter from her in the hospital mail, thanking me for all I had done. It didn't seem like I did anything.

Families filled with belief, a baby boy, a loved one's body, it seems there are these circles trying to close. Asking not for judgment, in orbits other than my own. Needing just to be themselves, and not like me.

ENCORE!!

One of the brightest moments in my career occurred when I worked in endoscopy. The patients had changing rooms and lockers that were private, but they were asked to wait in a line of chairs out in the open. As a result, there was no privacy for these semi-naked, starving (NPO) cleaned out (GI prep) souls who nervously waited to be sedated and have their various innards probed.

In the line of people was a man who was working up a head of steam about the wait. His physician had been called to an emergency, and so his bronchoscopy was well over an hour behind schedule. He had a long list of complaints: he had driven all the way from the Upper Peninsula, he hadn't had a blamed thing to eat, and no cigarettes or chew since last night, these doctors got paid to do a job and they should be doing it, and he wasn't going to wait one more minute. All this played to the audience at hand.

I began to console him as best I could. I pointed out that schedules can't always be kept and doctors have to work at putting out brush fires. We would give him a lot to drink and he could smoke after the test. And then, my personal favorite: he was as close to having this performed as he would ever be, having driven, fasted, abstained from tobacco. Why not wait just one hour more, or whatever it would take, to complete this test here and now, instead of packing up and running away, only to have to repeat the process?

The whole room was quiet for a moment, and then the other patients began to applaud. Two men, two women, in hospital pajamas, acknowledged my little speech. He didn't say anything, perhaps becoming aware of the others near him in like circumstances.

I don't know. It was pretty good reasoning, the part about being close to the finish line. And sadly, after this man's test, before he was fully awake, the doctor came from the room shaking his head, telling us that it really looked like cancer. But he'd send the specimens to know for sure.

Maybe the patient should have run. Or maybe he knew all along. But it was nice to hear applause for my little moment in the spotlight.

ADVICE TO NEW GRADS

- Look into their eyes. Say "hello" to your patients like there is nothing wrong and you're glad to see them. Even when they have weeping decubitus, or stool from their axilla to their great toe or horrible smelling mushrooms of tumor growing like cauliflower from a cancerous primary site. Even if their stomas are black or their feet are filled with gangrene, look into their eyes, and say, "Hello," to the person lost inside.

- "No" is a complete sentence. Try it. Say "no" when staffing calls you on your day off; when the charge nurse wants you to take both new admits; when patients keep holding the hoop higher and higher and you can't jump through it anymore. There is an answer. "No."

- I kiss some patients and hug even more. I flirt with women and men alike and never once have I been taken wrong. Maybe it's because I am nearing the age of 60 and who would take me seriously anyway?

- "Accurate I and O" means measuring all of the fluids going in and out. It doesn't mean you have to yell at the poor lady when she drops the toilet paper in the hat, even after the third time. I've performed some interesting experiments with toilet paper and water, using what I call the small, medium and large wad data. I doubt that my measurements have ever led to unnecessary treatments.

- Repeat after me, "I don't know." It's okay. I've done this for 25 years and I still can't work more than a few hours without saying it.

- Hold hands. With only a couple of exceptions, there is no excuse for wearing gloves to hold hands.

- Despite everything they tell you about this, sit on the bed. Act like you're going to stay for a while. Like you are not thinking of the blood sugar of the patient next door, or your break time. Listen. Sit and listen.

- Give more back rubs; take fewer vitals. It won't be long until you can recognize when someone's heart rate is up, blood pressure down and respirations labored, even from the door. The subtle color changes, the facial expressions, the work of breathing. *Then*, take vitals and skip the back rub. But mostly, the other way around is best.

- It is not okay to argue over your schedule, worry about your work load, your insignificant pay raise, or the other nurse who left the room in a mess, *in front of your patients*. Pretend they are paying for your help. Pretend they could have had anyone for their nurse, but they chose you.

- More and more, I find there is almost no reason for whispered, confidential reports at change of shift. Somehow, patients *know* how sick they are. They *know* they have been incontinent five times in eight hours. They *know* their husband hasn't come or called in three days. They even *know* when they've been a pain in the ass, though probably you'll want to word it a little differently when they can hear you. Maybe we should always talk about our patients as though they can hear us.

- I've told many of my patients that I'm no saint. When I'm giving them my little speech about no more smoking, drinking, being a couch potato or eating the fat off the pork chop. I try to let them know I've been there. Actually, I only need about an hour's notice before the end of the world. That should be enough time for a couple of cigarettes, a shot of Jim Beam and a hot fudge sundae in bed, of course.

- Find out what the absolute minimum amount of charting required by your institution is, and do that much and not a word more. Don't feel guilty that you work with others who write novels. If you've checked the square beside "dry and intact" under dressing, that's enough. Spend time elsewhere, looking up drugs, reading about some unfamiliar disease, or in the rooms of your patients.

- Everything is connected to everything else. Like a delicate string and balsa wood mobile, in perfect balance. Even a paper clip, dragging on just one part, makes the mobile go out of balance. So, if you think you are only into neuro or renal, if you just like cardiac care or post-partum moms, don't forget that it's all tied together and, often, the balance is what they need the most help with, not just one organ.

- Make your answers short. First, answer the question you think your patient is most worried about. Remember when that nice salesman came to your house and measured all your rooms and showed you all the carpet samples and padding for more than an hour and a half? Only at the end did he tell you that it would cost more than two grand. And you know exactly what your answer was. It's like that. Get to the point. Tell 'em how much it's going to cost.

- Don't be a flash in the pan. If you think you've got to get your master's degree and become director of nursing in the first year, you'll miss some of the fun. You can be a nurse for a long time. You'll need to grow *every* year, take classes, try new challenges. There will be times you won't want to learn anything new and times that you will. You'll do better in the long run if you don't try to cram for the final, especially when the course you're taking is called life.

A FEW REGRETS

When I was a very new nurse, I worked the afternoon shift on a surgical floor. One night, a very old man was trying to sleep but was quite restless because he was going to have a big surgery the next day.

I was in the room for another patient when he called me over to his bedside and asked me something I couldn't hear. I leaned closer, asked him to repeat it, and again, couldn't tell what it was. Finally, the third time, in a much louder voice he asked, "Can I squeeze your tittie?"

I was shocked and told him sternly, "No," and that if he continued to speak inappropriately I would have to get my supervisor.

My regret is that I didn't keep it light, that I didn't use humor. I could have said that only my husband got to do that, but I would keep him in mind if I ever became available.

This would not be the only time I would see people decompensate and loose their footing when facing the fear of illness or death.

ALL YOU NEED IS LOVE

The late '60s were dicey times to be young. We were supposed to rail against the establishment by burning our bras. I don't know, I suppose those bras that looked like armor and you were about to burst into a Wagner Opera, holding a shield and spear, maybe those should have been burned. But then some of my friends thought we should go braless, and wear band aids over our nipples. This is the sort of thing you can bring yourself to do only once. Youch!

About this time, there were groups of women that thought you should become more familiar with your Inner Goddess by using a mirror (and presumably a flashlight) to look at your cervix, becoming more aware of the womb. Even when I was more lithe and limber and weighed much less, this would have been quite a feat.

DOG SEX

My son Rob began to wonder out loud about sex last evening while we were walking our dog, Casey. Casey was approached by another male dog and they began the universal dog handshake, each sniffing the other's rear end to say "hello." After wondering why they did this and then thinking back to the time he had seen one dog on top of another, Rob opened up the perfect way for me to explain reproduction.

I drew comparisons between humans and dogs, but his questions seemed more focused on how dogs "do it," rather than people. "Why did we have Casey's balls cut off?" he wondered. Because the dog had been making a pest of himself almost daily by trying to impregnate the leg of your brother, I explained.

This made Rob choke with giggles. "Scott's little leggy-weggy was supposed to have puppywuppies, Casey?" he taunted as he patted the dog's head. Casey looked up at him with confused appreciation. Fortunately, Rob's brother was not on this walk.

Another area of particular interest was how the sperm and the egg each have one arm and one leg, one eye, which he surmised from my very brief explanation of genetics. I told him about menstruation. He wanted to know if girl dogs wore panties to catch the blood. I said, "Some do." (Even now, 30 years later, I get a little embarrassed when I remember our dachshund, before we had her fixed, in my mom's nice clean house, wearing these little plaid suspender things with a few Kleenexes tucked in.)

"How does the penis know not to pee when it decides to make sperm?" came next. And, "Why do boy dogs with no balls still sniff each other?"

Not only was I unable to answer his questions, I was also unable to get him back to human reproduction. Like how people can decide not to have babies, or why two people should be married first before they get on top of each other. All areas that interest parents and make kids go glassy-eyed or giggle.

HOW TO DEAL WITH DIFFICULT PEOPLE

No one likes angry people. They cause untold problems in the workplace and take up far too much of a manager's day. When tension mounts, brush fires erupt, and people close to the anger get burned: the incident report that is used to tell someone off, the abrupt phone calls or lectures in the hall.

What can you do? What antidote is available to neutralize the power these people wield over you? There are four things that can help:

1) Try having some insight into why they are difficult;

2) Try letting go of the rope;

3) Remember that both of you may need to agree to disagree;

4) And, recognize that it's almost never just about you.

I did a lot of on-call work for Hospice and many nights I was called out multiple times. Some problems were real and some were not. Our organization was used and abused by people who knew we were soft-hearted and would come.

Friday nights were the worst. One Friday night, I was driving to another county, had already been to one death, was driving to the next, had answered page after page about pain and nausea and bowels turned to cement, and then this doctor called demanding that I come right away to admit a dying patient he was sending home from the hospital to die. "It is his last wish," he pleaded and demanded.

I decided this was an excellent time to tell someone off. I wondered why his patient's health had so taken him by surprise that he could not have foreseen the need for our agency before this. I wondered about the trauma of an ambulance ride for a desperately ill person, who might easily die en route. I asked if he knew about the mountain of paperwork I would put the family through just to be able to sign him on, taking them away from the precious few minutes they might still have with their loved one. There was more, but he had lost interest and hung up.

It didn't matter that some of my lecture was true or right. What mattered was that I *was* Hospice for that phone call, and all the others. I got the Monday morning lecture. We were a small agency and needed patients. It was true this doctor routinely called on Fridays with "emergencies." And we learned that the patient in question had died within hours of the phone call, at the hospital.

At first, I saw this as proof, as ammunition for my case. And then, just hours into my shift on Monday, I realized what had happened. Somehow, I had become a monster.

The pager, the lack of sleep, the difficult, emotional work I was doing had changed me into a person who was glad to hear of someone's death to prove a point. Maybe I could have just said no to

had to adjust to post-partum stays that were often shorter than the labors themselves.

"We'll be doing drive-through deliveries," she said to me after she attended yet another meeting about cost containment. And, though there have always been teenagers having babies, children having children, she was surprised to see so many now, after her long time away.

Even if she isn't leading the pack yet, she has become a well-trained member of our OB staff. I congratulate the manager who hired her and our hospital for looking beyond the apparent void in her resume.

Compared to some of the most recently hired nurses, her resume looks empty. After all, she has not been working on her master's degree, though she received her BSN with honors years ago. She has not attended numerous conferences and in-services and she hasn't been chasing the paper tiger all these years, missing all the changes in documentation.

But look what she *has* been doing. Her family of two boys and three girls spans the third grade to college sophomore. For these beautiful children, she has sewn the fairy princess costume, baked Kermit the Frog cakes and attended every football game since her sons began to play. She has been room mom, Sunday school mom and lunch-room mom which, if you have ever done it, you know entitles her to the Purple Heart.

She has taken care of sore throats, chicken pox times five, broken wrists and ankles. She has lived through three puberties. She has done the books for her husband's business, and they are still married.

Piece of cake? There was never an orientation for this important work, though her family set a good example. Certainly there was no pay. Not even when one of her babies, fretful and sick, made her stay up all night walking the floors.

She had to do most of the work alone. Most of the decisions couldn't wait. She had to know, somehow, what to do when the refrigerator stopped making things freeze. She was supposed to know when to take her kids to the doctor, when to stay home, how to handle the awkward problem of the teacher who picks on your kid, but lives one house away. And what to do when both pairs of shoes were left out in the rain. And when the economy went belly up, and nobody wanted to buy boats from her husband's marina, she had to know how to cut costs, and explain it to the kids just before Christmas.

There was no one else to call when she was sick. At times her work was lonely. When she felt unappreciated, lost in the repetitive maze of wash, fold, wash again, there was never another adult female to bolster her failing self-esteem.

And so I congratulate the bosses where I work. Sometimes, I picture that I am the boss and I have just interviewed her and offered her a nursing position. I don't say, "We'll give you a chance and see if you can make it." Instead I hear myself saying, "We are honored that you have decided on us as your employer. Your varied experiences and talents will add much to our organization. Here, won't you sit down and let me get you a cup of coffee?"

My friend will do well. Her hard work is no dream. We have everything to gain. I wish her a smooth transition and warm welcome.

LATE SIGNS

Sometimes people are so sick and they stay in the hospital too long. Too long is when the men are doing beer ads and the women are making the sign of the beaver. These both are very bad. The patient has given up and may never get better, psychologically or physically.

When a man can't reach his Kleenex box or ice water or adjust his pillow, even though nothing whatever was done to his arms or hands, he has "fallen and he can't reach his beer."

When a woman no longer cares who looks between her legs and, even when family is there, just lets it all hang out, that is the sign of the beaver. She has been in a freefall to the point that even about this she doesn't care.

35

MARY AND LEROY

I first met Mary ten minutes before her baby was born. Her husband, Leroy, hovered over her, his small body dwarfed by Mary's rather expansive frame. The focal point was Mary's bulging perineum – and the head of the baby pushing its way into the world.

"Mary, open your legs," the doctor urged. Leroy repeated into her ear, "Mary, open up, buttercup." Shaking and crying, Mary said, "I'm afraid, I'm afraid." Then, Mary shifted her weight, parted her legs and her daughter Hannah was born.

"I knew you could do it!" Leroy exclaimed, as he kissed her over and over. Short and wiry, Leroy wore a sleeveless cut-off sweatshirt that made his leathery skin and many tattoos hard to miss – the pale red rose encircling his navel, for example. Though almost completely bald, he still had enough hair to gather into a ponytail at the back, sticking through the hole in a duckbilled cap emblazoned with, "The Right Stuff."

In time, I came to think of both Leroy and Mary as truly the right stuff. Mary, 22, had been married to 56-year old Leroy for six years, her second marriage, his sixth. "It's working," she told me later. "Probably 'cause with all his marriages, he understands women real good." The difference in their ages meant little. Mary was wise beyond her years and Leroy – an old hand at fatherhood –

wept with joy like a first-time daddy. He choked out, "God, I love you, Mary!"

After the baby was taken to the nursery, Mary righted herself, fear forgotten, and began making simple demands: first for a soft drink and then some tissue. "Sure babe," Leroy said, handing her tissues while edging toward the door. "And take Momma with you," she added. The quiet figure huddled in the corner came to life and struggled to stand. A slightly smaller replica of Mary, she wore dark glasses and used a cane. Her scalp showed palely beneath her dry, thinning hair. She looked to be about 60. When I'd first seen the trio I thought this woman and Leroy were Mary's parents.

"I can't go nowhere till I have my shot," her mother said to no one in particular. She rummaged in her purse, brought out a vial of insulin and a syringe, pulled down the waistband of her pants and injected herself in the abdomen. That accomplished, she snapped her pants back into place, turned to me, and announced: "I'm gonna need something to eat or I'll probably pass out on you..."

Before I could give my lecture about caring for the patient, and visitors would have to... Mary told her mother point-blank, "Get outta here, Momma. Don't go bothering the nurse. For God's sake, Leroy, take her to the cafeteria." As Momma shuffled past the bed, Mary explained,

"She's got sugar. It's screwed up her eyes and feet – she's just 36."

With her family off on errands, Mary directed her requests to me. "I want my baby. How soon can I have Hannah?" "Right now," I told her, and went to get her darling new daughter. While I was gone, Mary combed her hair and replaced her hospital gown with a shimmering black negligee.

"I sell lingerie on the side," she told me, no doubt in response to the look I must have given her when I returned. Barely an hour after delivery, Mary decided that she was ready to move to a regular room. When I suggested a wheelchair ride, she replied, "Hell no, I feel great!" I found a hospital gown to throw over her shoulders and we paraded down the hall together, bassinet in tow, when Mary spotted the scale.

"Oh, gee, let's see how much I lost," she said happily as she stepped up. There, for all to see, was the balance at 274. "Boy, Hannah didn't 'mount to a hill of beans, but 'course I do retain water..." she announced. I was thinking she retained a lot more than water as we got her settled into her room. There, she took on her baby's care with a vengeance. It hadn't even crossed her mind that anyone else would watch over her little "rosebud."

The next day, though, Mary's day of discharge, I found her with the curtain pulled and her head hanging. Still wearing her black negligee,

Mary sported hot pink fingernails and rose and lavender eye shadow.

"What's up, Mary?" I asked, thinking of the larger-than-life persona of yesterday. "Oh, I don't know, just tired, I guess."

"You know, even with a fine delivery and great baby, you're entitled to feel a little depressed afterward," I said, hoping I was offering her the flag of surrender she might need. She did. Tears began to roll down her cheeks, and out came her story and the complexities of her very special life.

Hannah was the second baby she'd had after artificially inseminating herself. Long before she and Leroy met, he had had penile cancer and, in those days, as Mary put it, "they cut the whole thing off, just in case." Leroy and Mary "did real good" with alternative forms of lovemaking, but making babies was another matter. So using one of her mother's insulin syringes, Mary collected Leroy's semen and "stuck it up there just right, 'xactly on my hot day."

"Hot day?" I asked.

"Yeah, you know, when the mucus from your cervix makes a long string, she explained. This new mom knew a lot.

"So you and Leroy didn't go to some fancy clinic, but just did the insemination at home?"

"Yup! Right in Ellsworth, U.S.A."

Before long, we were gossiping like old friends. Mary told me they had two sons at home, one by Leroy via the syringe who was five years old and one who was nine years old and fathered by her first husband. Any way you cut it, this woman got started early. She told me that her first marriage ended in divorce because he used to beat both her and the child. Now she lived in peace and loved Leroy and her growing family.

I had almost forgotten why I'd come to see her in the first place. "Mary, in all of this I haven't heard you tell me why you're down today," I asked. "It's Hannah. Do you think she looks jaundiced? I'm scared she might have something wrong with her liver." She told me.

First, I assured her Hannah was fine, and then I told her I was impressed by her knowledge. She told me she wanted to become a midwife someday and that she had passed the exam to get her high school diploma. I told her she would make a great midwife and that she was wise beyond her years.

As I got up to go, she added one last thing – her only acknowledgement that her life was anything out of the ordinary. "Ya know, a long time ago, my best friend told me not to look at other people to see if I'm okay, but just keep lookin' inside my own head."

Silenced by her wisdom, I stood there thoughtfully until the door opened with Leroy, bursting in, "Is my Buttercup ready to go?" I assured him, she was.

Sometimes when I see a large woman in the store, with a baby in her grocery cart, I hope it will be Mary. I meant to get her address and I forgot to give her a hug. If she could have stayed longer, I think she could have taught me a lot more.

ONLY IN AMERICA

A nurse friend of mine does mission work in Nicaragua for two weeks each year. She assists in a MASH tent helping the surgeons who also make the trip. People sometimes walk as much as three days to come for help. Once there, they might wait one, two, even three days, fasting, in line for possible surgery.

A mother of twelve had a badly inflamed prolapsed uterus. She was anesthetized, given one dose of antibiotic, had her hysterectomy, rested one day on the mats her family brought with them, and then walked home. No pain killers after the first day.

In today's mail, I received three months worth of pills for my stomach, depression and arthritis. I had, completely free to me, a mammogram, bone scan, colonoscopy and stress cardiolyte during this year. Also a series of lab work and a few office visits. The last time I saw my physician I went because of sore heels. He thoughtfully taught me some stretching exercises but, as I walked to my car, I felt a little short-changed. My heels still hurt; wasn't it more of a medical emergency?

Possibly, the real problem for my feet is the 40-plus pounds of fat I should get rid of. My doctor was kind enough not to mention this. I pay a small fee at our local college so I can leave my house in my car, drive to this beautiful workout gym and try to keep my strength up and my weight under control.

I have lost only one day of work because of pain – the day before my root canal. I would not recommend this as a choice of leisure activity, but I feel blessed to have dental care available. In everything I have done this year, no disease was found. Yet more than $5,000 was spent by my employer's insurance company to confirm this or maintain my health with my prescriptions.

I am so blessed - so spoiled by my American life. I have a job in a high unemployment economy. This is good work in a beautiful town. I feel cared for by my co-workers and valued by my managers. My patients tell me I do a good job and sometimes give us chocolates to help with weight gain.

My husband and I have been saving for a long time – believing that, some day, no matter who is in the White House, the check will *not* be in the mail.

My retirement problems are not exactly my employer's fault. Everyone is living longer, taking up more benefits promised to them. Behind every GM car sticker is a huge, ever-growing, cost of retirement benefits that make it harder and harder to compete. One analyst said GM was a retirement company that happens to make cars on the side.

Our medical dollars are so precarious now that they have become a cake walk. Remember the child's game of the missing chair? When the music stops, the person left standing is out. In good conscience, I don't want to retire and take the last dollar from my hospital's dwindling funds. We need health care in the future and that may mean changing the way benefits are figured. I sure don't have the answers; maybe no one does.

One place to start is by making your own list of all the benefits you have in your life, personal and work. I have worked a lot of places and never have found one like this. To me, it is the best. I feel grateful every day to work here.

But even if you disagree and believe we are not paid enough, given enough say in patient care, have poor retirement benefits and have to contribute too much for healthcare, at the very least we are still living in a country where it is okay to say so.

I often wonder what the mother from Nicaragua would think if she were to come to our hospital.

Sometimes, when you put your hand into the candy jar and try to grab too much, your fist is too full to pull back out. And only in America would we not see that we could have enough candy if only we would let go.

PEDAL TO THE METAL

During the last few weeks, I have been precepting EMTs through their required ICU experience. They are on their way to paramedic ratings and studying for the Advanced Cardiac Life Support (ACLS) exam. Precepting is teaching them their basics but this experience must seem like a bad dream. One filled with comatose patients lost beneath tubes and lines and the sound of blips and beeps and muffled horns.

On the first orientation night, they each have soft-scared eyes filled with awe and fear of the unknown. And, as if to complicate it more, beyond the vents and pumps and bags filled with urine or blood or bile, the old-guard, long-time ICU nurses humble them with looks of "who-the-hell-are-you?"

Year after year, these nurses are willing to give expert care to patients, but are known to eat their young. It somehow comforts me that they are as cold to all newcomers as they are to my EMTs.

The real lesson I must teach is not so much technology but self esteem. These gentlemen of the wailing siren know it is whispered that they are really only glorified truck drivers. They need much convincing that they are worthwhile and not too stupid to learn. But in this ICU there is so much for them to comprehend.

They do a lot more CPR than we do, in part because we see the impending death and deal with the changes almost as they happen with medications, fluids and other therapies. They must take things as they are: crushed bodies in collapsed cars, clothing that must be cut off, a vein that must be found. They try to bring someone back to life and try to drive the truck fast enough.

Most of them smoke and are overweight. But, on the whole, they are big and strong. There is a duck-billed cap on one and a large belt buckle embossed with a jumping white tail deer in relief. Snapped to their belts are their radios and leather pouches with every kind of tool.

They follow me around like a shadow. I have to be careful not to step backward because they are always there. Sometimes they sit next to me at the desk and climb into their chair by lifting one leg over the back. And when we go to supper (dinner was what they had at lunch) they confide their stories to me. The wife that split, the kids they love, the hopes and dreams of improving themselves. These are mostly local boys with high school diplomas. Each hopes for a buck this fall, now that the wood is stacked and the plastic is on the windows.

They order meat with gravy and mashed potatoes and Jell-O and pie. They drink their coffee with the spoon still in the cup, swinging it out of the way with one finger, their hand surrounding the cup. All this at two a.m.

They seem to love me. And I love them. We've been through a lot. Our patients have died. And when they haven't, we were tortured with the possibility that they might. Through it all, I've tried hard to make them feel important, to remind them that they are helping even when they don't understand.

Of course death is not new to them. Nor blood and guts. But weeping loved ones are a painful new dimension. One EMT thoroughly studied his shoes as I began to help one weeping family. He cleared his throat and walked purposefully to the door and through it, closing it gently behind him. I was left with the hysterical wife and sobbing son. He was trapped for the duration in the bathroom.

Some have had years of on-the-road experience. Others are quite new and young. Bob was somewhere in between. But, even with all the time in the world, some things are still missed. After the first set of vitals and assessment one night, things seemed to settle into a pleasant routine. I asked Bob to go ahead and do the next set of vitals and assessment without my help, but to be sure and include a rectal temp as I knew this to be much more accurate. Off he went, only to return five minutes later to get me. "I can't find it," he whispered. "What, Bob?" I asked. He looked pale and I knew our conversation must continue out of the earshot of others. A few steps away, I learned it was the rectum he couldn't find. "I've never seen one before," he confessed.

I thought of lots of one-liners: "Seen one, seen 'em all," but instead we took a flashlight and had a good look, agreeing afterwards that it was pretty dark down there. None of this was within hearing of the patient or other nurses.

Kevin was my student of intractable math. He could do it all right, even get correct answers, but he quite literally didn't know what he had when he finished. He kept asking about the drip factor, a way of counting the number of drips per minute that certain tubing provides, to help know how much and fast a fluid is running in.

We *never* use this tubing with calculated drips. Running dopamine or epinephrine in this kind of tubing, with the potential for it to become "wide-open," courts homicide. I told Kevin this. He could take the patient's weight, convert it into kilograms and figure out the number of micrograms per kilogram per minute, which is a little complicated. But he would always ask me, "What about the drip factor?" He was immobilized. It kept him back.

Finally, I dusted off a little lie and made it into legend. "Kevin," I told him, "I too had this same problem years ago, and my instructor had her hands full. I kept thinking drip factor should be figured in. So one day, shortly before my final exam, she did me a big favor. She said, 'Katie, fuck the drip factor.' And I did great on that test. So

Kevin, my advice to you is..." He finished my sentence for me. He looked away. He'd lost permission to ask his favorite question. But a week from now, all 12 EMTs must pass the math test to stay in the program. And some of them will certainly have to put the pedal to the metal in study time.

I want them all to pass. Each is a wonderful, caring man. And all they will have achieved, if they become paramedics, is a hard job, long hours and low pay. I suspect each of them would do this work for almost nothing. How *do* you compensate someone who gets bitten by the family dog, slogs through snow drifts up to his armpits to get to the car with the two belligerent drunks in it, or delivers a baby in the back seat of a car?

PLAYING GOD

Sometimes when Charlie flies us downstate from Harbor Springs to Jackson late at night, I ask him to put Alma or Lansing on the right so I can see the places that have been a part of my history. Clear landmarks tell the locations: the white spire of the chapel at Alma College where I went to school.

I remember helping to substitute the taped sound of the tolling bells in the Chapel with "Louie, Louie!" It turned out the length of time it took to ring out 12 noon on Parents Sunday just about covered the whole song!

And when we are over Lansing, I can see the capitol building and imagine that I am looking in the window of the church across from it, into the dark interior to see the light of the candle always burning in the red glass holder. Ten thousand feet up, it seems I could fall out and over the wing, head over heels to the ground safely, to stand by that window. I would look in at the pew that held my mom and dad on the Sundays I was baptized, confirmed, married and when my sons were baptized, all at this church. And as I stood there on tiptoe, my feet would be touching the ground above my sister and dad whose ashes are buried by the ancient brick wall that bears witness to so much that is important in my life.

Such contrasting and conflicting images remind me that I try to play God by commanding whole towns to move left or right; and then I humbly beg for something in my prayers. I attend the Episcopal Church here where the ancient words of the service seem to heal me: tender mercies, manifold sins and propitiation for them. All words from my childhood I still cannot define, but understand all the same.

I occasionally rope Charlie into going with me. He sits quietly, listening to the "show" and we drive home in silence, knowing better than to debate. On rare occasions, I tell him I believe in the Trinity and he tells me he does too. His being three indestructible laws of nature: the acceleration of gravity, (9.8 meters per second per second),

Ohm's Law (not just a good idea, it's the law) which is voltage = amperes x resistance and finally, the Bernoulli Principle: an increase in velocity occurs simultaneously with a decrease in pressure. These three keep his feet on the ground, his radios working and his airplane in the air.

This is usually the time he also mentions he doesn't have to tithe or listen to talks about the trinity or, for that matter, even believe in them. They go right on being true, regardless of what anyone may choose to believe. In this at least we agree. There *is* a power greater than ourselves, providing watchful care no matter what.

PSEUDONYM

I have been bitten by the wasp I work for but am coming along nicely after pulling out the offending stinger, looking it over carefully, and seeing that it doesn't belong to me. My boss "Marilyn," was not pleased that the American Journal of Nursing wanted to print my story and told me I needed to run it by administration so she could feel "comfortable." And, while she didn't know what I had been doing in the ICU room I had just walked out of ten minutes before (CPR on a progressive corpse), this suddenly was important to her. I found it hard to control myself and keep her comfort in mind.

I told her the administration was welcome to oversee my nursing but I could not seek their approval for my writing. Marilyn countered with the suggestion that, if only a few things were changed in my article, then it would not offend anybody and didn't I want it that way? This opened up one of my favorite themes: how unfortunate it is when our only goal in life is to stay exactly in the middle. We lose the really high points in the human experience.

Her eyes glazed over and, in the distance, just twenty feet or so away, I could see the weeping family of the patient who had just died. I felt emboldened. I knew I was right. People are alive at the beginning of the shift and dead at the end. Who needs the middle? Why not make waves, even unfriendly ones?

So on I went: I told her about my not wanting to always be the same, just to vote Republican, get a brush-cut, drive a sedan, please everyone. Now her eyes were dilated and fixed.

We drifted off. I agreed she could pass the manuscript along to management. If it became published in a national journal it would hardly go unnoticed. I called the Journal in New York and they were very kind and agreed to my use of a pseudonym. I thought a lot about this. Kept me busy for a while, thinking and thinking. Then I hit upon the idea of using Marilyn's name...

♂ RN

I like men in nursing. Right away, I know there is a risk in identifying a group as somehow better or worse. Affirmative action is supposed to mean that you interview a prospective employee while blindfolded and with earplugs and still pick a member of a struggling minority. Even so, I like men, and I really like them in nursing.

Our hospital has a lot of them. Something about the fishing and hunting, the stacks of wood beside the log cabin, the mystique of living in northern Michigan seems to attract them. They stay. They build homes with their own hands, bow hunt, buy boats with monthly payments due through 2019. They work hard at being nurses. No better, no worse, they deliver excellent care to our patients.

But the real reasons I like men in nursing are as follows.

Because of Bob. Upon returning from vacation he was greeted warmly and shortly began bragging about how he had potty-trained his young son. We had expected to hear about game trophies, but he didn't really mention any of that. He had gotten nowhere with the M&M incentive program, but what finally worked were frozen colored-water ice cubes in the toilet. His little son could take aim. And, even in this, Bob had to brag at what a good aim his progeny had inherited from him.

Because of Tom. Besides teaching me EKG rhythms and more than I'll ever want to know about hemi-blocks and widening QRSs, he also taught me that it's okay for men to cry. His dog died after he had tried desperately to nurse him back to health. Tom knew the time had come. He'd taken home discarded egg-crate mattress pads to comfort the arthritic joints of his dog's aged bones. There were countless trips to the vet and trials of pain medications, but the dog still cried with position changes. When he couldn't even eat a tuna sandwich and no longer could wag hello, Tom put a butterfly needle in the dog's forearm and did the last kind thing he could.

Because of Dick. Good old reliable Dick, sitting at the front desk, making out assignments. I would say in a loud voice, "So how's my favorite Pollack," when I arrived at work. A noncommittal grunt was his answer, along with, "I think I'll give *this* assignment to Katie." Supposedly the worst, but really it wasn't. He never asked us to do more than he would do, and did. There's probably nothing Dick hasn't seen. Years of emergency room work in a large Detroit hospital honed his skills, but all the same he has his tender side.

One time I asked Dick what was wrong with Sue, another nurse who seemed to have grown sullen. Instead of joining me in some conspiratorial conversation, he said, "Nothing wrong with Sue that wouldn't be wrong with you if your son just got sent to the Gulf." Or of a new grad: "She needs our support. I don't care if she did or didn't do something wrong. She'll be a damn good nurse only if we encourage her." With Dick, it's not okay to gossip. He should give lessons.

And because of Bill. I have watched or helped him give enemas to female patients in their eighties with more dignity and gentleness than many female co-workers.

Because of Jeff. Maybe because he is the father of three little women. I don't know, but I count Jeff as my friend. Not my male friend. Just friend. I like to talk with him because of the human being that he is. Sometimes he comes around the corner and grabs my shoulder and gives it a squeeze, particularly when he knows I'm stressed or working hard. And it slows me down, even if only for a minute. And I think more squeezes and hugs should be given, I know my patients need them. So do nurses.

When I work with men, I don't spend as much time talking about my menstrual cycle and how to get the baked-on lasagna out of the pan. It's nice to have men around. Even with the talk of cars, the deer rifle controversy, "No, I still go for the lever action, you can take the bolt..." And yes, Ken is a changed man when he gets his limit of blue gills.

Just when I am supposed to be learning the politically correct way to talk of race, age and sex, when hymnals must have "mankind" replaced with "humankind," there are risks in saying "I like men." I just do. Every thinking person knows there's a difference between men and women, and those differences do not stop when people become registered nurses. That's the part I like the most.

SCREAM

Something in my friend's goodbye last night frightened me. We were at the reception for her second marriage. It was a lovely evening, really. But when she walked us to the door to say goodbye, there was a strange but familiar look in her eyes. It reminded me of a three-year old being left on a Sunday morning at church school. Even after the nursery door has closed, the parents can hear their child scream.

We knew her first husband and the four of us had gone through the rites of passage of our twenties together. In small apartments, we gave fondue parties with the equipment we acquired at our weddings. Our furniture was from the Salvation Army, the floors were covered with orange shag rugs. We drank to excess and laughed and smoked cigarettes; we thought we were grown up. Our jobs were new just after college and Vietnam. We moved around without encumbrances, no diaper bags to weigh us down. Our egos were large with the effort of pushing out of our teens, leaving parents, getting through school, getting that first job. But we were fickle and, when our employers didn't please us, we went elsewhere to make our way. It seemed our futures were only limited by the numbers of copies we could make of our résumés.

Now, our self-esteem is shrinking. We are less attractive and downright meaner. If we skipped an election years ago because we failed to register, now we are flaming, dyed-in-the-wool Republicans or Democrats and it seems impossible to spend an evening with the couple next door or family members of a different stripe. Just what we loved before, being free of family, having nothing to hold us back, going from job to job, now scares the hell out of us. Our address book has names that are lined out; the people that we loved have died. We are plagued by loneliness. A chronic bitter pill we daily swallow reminding us of all the losses, all the wrong turns and mishaps of our lives.

Our friend has cast her fate with this new husband. She shows him like some trophy she has won. She wants us to see the drawings of the house they plan to build. I assume this new husband makes much more than number one did. I wonder at the emphasis here.

There is a line from a movie in which Barbra Streisand plays a hooker. She is confronted by the wife of one of her regular clients. Understandably, the wife is angry. Barbra says to her in almost a collegial way, "We all lift our skirts for a price." This wisdom does not escape me. I too have made a deal with my husband, and we have slowly arrived at some kind of synergy. We have agreed: this is how we will live together, this is what we need from each other. If you want to grow old with me, here is the price.

My friend is lonely. I should know. I was with her when her first husband died of cancer. The first to hug her, give her a glass of water, a tissue, coffee. She was too young to stay single for long.

But what was it that I saw in her eyes last night? Some request to give our blessing on her marriage? Her new house? Their future? Some show that we will relinquish our memories of her first husband and take up with the new? Congratulations that they both escaped the abyss of loneliness? And for what they give to one another, will it fill the empty space the ticking clock has made?

Was that what I saw?

Oh friend, dear friend, bless you. Bless this new husband and Godspeed. Run from this pain I think I understand. Go now to your future, bright with hope. Because in all of us, no matter how great or good our fortune, there is that silent scream.

SETPOINT

The human body is funny about feeling comfortable. We like to be at 98.6 degrees

Fahrenheit in a 70-degree room. And the reason we feel cold when we're actually getting a fever is that the distance between the two has been increased. So, even though the room is still at 70 degrees, it feels much colder with every degree of temperature *we* increase. It's all a matter of variation from our setpoint.

There is a setpoint in the rest of our life, but sometimes it is buried deeply in our psyche. If we grew up with a domineering father or demanding mother, we quite often surround ourselves with similar people in our friends, lovers and spouses.

If we know we are short on money with bills mounting and no income in sight, quite often we do the worst thing possible by buying things we least need to make it feel okay, to somehow return to the feeling we had when things seemed normal.

Counterintuitive. We do the things we ought not do, and don't do the things we should. Just because of brain chemistry, or some well-remembered neuronal synapse that tells us we are in familiar territory, that our choice is right because it connects in some way with a setpoint, even from long ago.

A woman marries an abusive husband. And though she doesn't know it, this reminds her of a parent who regularly used a strap to mete out punishment for wrong-doing. A man knows he must not feel, not because he doesn't, but because in all the time he knew his father, he never saw him cry.

Over and over, we try to blame the thermostat on the wall to keep the temperature around us the same distance from our own, never guessing that we might be febrile. Never guessing that success in life might mean that we have to change our long believed setpoint.

THE LORD'S PRAYER

I went to France when I was in college, years ago. In Paris at the time, there were metal circular shelters of a sort, with a drain in the floor, right out on the sidewalks, and they were supposed to be restrooms. You could see feet and pushed-down pants below the metal screen. I know Americans are obsessed with toilet issues and we bathe a lot more than most cultures, but these crude toilets were almost more than I could stand.

Our bus tour was leaving and I absolutely had to pee. I stood there and stood there willing myself to do that very thing. But I could not. My travel companion helpfully said over and over in a loud voice, "Come on! Come on!" Any thought of blending in, becoming invisible, was lost. Finally, she suggested I say the Lord's Prayer. To calm down, I guess. And I'm happy to report somewhere between bread and trespass, there were results.

THE LOVE LETTER

Sometimes I can hardly stand to be in the same room with you. At night, after supper you fall asleep with the TV blaring. Your snoring is in syncopation with *The Simpsons*, your favorite show, and I think: our lives have been reduced to this? A real-life rerun of *The Honeymooners*? What did I expect? The reading of a sonnet, dozens of roses, a five-course dinner?

When we do tasks together, our differences flash like fire between us. I, the generalist, you the left-brained detail person. Each of us thinking, "Oh no! She/he is going to do it that way?" We roll up our sleeves and begin the task. You completely wash and dry two squares of linoleum while I wash all the rest of the kitchen, hall and bath. I should have known you were this way before we married. I came to your apartment to help before a party. I cleaned and did the food, two loads of laundry, and you alphabetized your record album collection.

What did we first see in each other? What magnet drew us close? The sexuality that once consumed us has withered. Your ears I once played with provocatively are now the source of constant grooming. When we undress I see we have gained a pound for every year of marriage. But as a nurse, I know we look like many of the patients I see. We are the norm.

How can my life have come to this? Sometimes I look at you and think only of escape. I imagine taking the dog and driving west. We would travel to Utah or Arizona and hole up in a motel. My hair is long and cascades down my back, I am 30 lbs. lighter and my ankles are not swollen. When I go across the street to the saloon for dinner, a cowboy asks me to dance. He is polite and, as he wraps his arm around my shoulder to lead me to the center of the wooden floor, I smell his aftershave, the warmth of his body, and the leather of his boots. And whiskey. He swirls me around the floor, displaying me like some prize. Later, he smells a lot more like whiskey than all the rest. Much later, I realize that my dog will hate living out of a car, my money will run out and I will cry myself to sleep at night longing for home and family and you. And somehow my cowboy and saloon out west have gained me nothing and I am nowhere, but far away from where I need to be.

Today, we are to meet for lunch. As I wait and watch the people walking in from the parking lot, I look for your distinctive bowlegged walk. And when I see you in the distance, I feel something in me jump. My heart? Something of welcome and recognition, of home and familiarity and rescue.

You greet me with a warm hug, a kiss and "Hi, Honey!" never suspecting I have come home from dancing with cowboys. My hair is barber short, all 30 pounds are reattached. You seem so glad to see me. Unaware. Liking me, loving me. You tell me some story important to you, with the face of a child whose turn has come for show and tell. I try to listen and hope you will not ask about the faraway look in my eyes.

I remember your enduring kindness to me; sometimes just your patient silence as you helped me live with mental illness. I remember your tears when our sons were born and irrevocably changed our lives forever. To see these small creatures in your arms with the glitter of emotion in your eyes was something I will never forget. Yet sometimes even now, I see you cup a hapless bug in your hand and carry it to the door to freedom and I see the same gentleness and caring. One time you stopped the car on a country road to take a small turtle from the middle to the side of the road. Hissing and spitting, he tried to cross again.

I know mushy love confuses you. I have known your parents for too long not to realize feelings were not discussed and rarely demonstrated in your childhood. But you were a quick study, and came to hugs and love words.

Sometimes, I think you are the only one I can tell something to, the repository of all my history and the only other living person who speaks the language only you and I know. You will do anything for me, as I will for you. Of course, this comes with loud remonstrations and trailing arguments but, in the end, we each always win. Maybe because having our way is almost always, also each other's.

You have swallowed the bitter with the sweet. I feel like some inedible plant that poisons all but one animal species: you. And you are sometimes inspiration in reverse: you make me work to be the person you are not. I grow stronger living with you purely from the irritation.

More often, though, I wish I could be like you. You are so innocent, less critical than I. You don't even see the stuff I do, sweetly ignorant. You do not blame. I'm high maintenance, inflexible, and bear no resemblance to the dancing girl of my dreams, pulling back her long red hair.

And yet you love me. And I love you. I don't understand this odd outcome. For all that we are not, or have lost to time, you comfort me.

How could my life have come to this? I thank God every day that it has.

THE PLOT

My uncle-in-law Gordy has a thriving business in "pet planting" as he affectionately calls it. After two or three martinis, he tells embellished stories of his "calling" to bury the well-loved dogs and cats and occasional guinea pigs of St. Paul, Minnesota.

He doesn't exactly say he's a member of the Better Business Bureau, but I gather his grief-stricken patrons trust him completely. As they hand him their dead pets and write checks for 50 dollars, they see only Pastor Gordy, as some of his repeat business call him. There in the small front office of the mortuary, which is really the 12-by-60 foot trailer he hauled to the site and which for them is the gate to animal heaven, is an area adorned with sachets of catnip and dog biscuits.

As they make their tearful farewells, the patrons can choose from a variety of memorial jewelry that will forever preserve a locket of the deceased's fur. Then Gordy arranges a time for the service and, as the owners pulls away in their car, he takes the dearly departed to the rear door of the trailer. There, depending on its state of rigor, he reduces the animal to a compressed, cylindrical shape.

By breaking the bones (if necessary) with a large mallet he keeps hanging on some twine near the back door, Gordy can usually get cats to be "no bigger than a quart of milk" and large dogs can be "about the size of four paint cans, stacked one on another."

Then with a post-hole digger, he "slips them in real nice," slaps the sod back down and puts the plastic flowers over the top. When the owners return for the funeral, he reads Scripture, Kahlil Gibran, or something from *Field and Stream*. He always invites them to come back any time to visit their pet's resting place.

Gordy hopes they don't all come at once. As near as he can figure, he will be able to fit about five thousand dogs and cats in the one-acre park. With guinea pigs mixed in, probably more.

THE REAL RIGHT STUFF

Recently, my alma mater wrote asking me to return to school this fall for homecoming. I wrote them back the following letter:

Dear Alma College:
      This letter is in regard to your frequent mailings and phone calls that query me about my alum status. Let's be honest, they are really about wanting me to send money.
      If I had a lot of money, I would direct it elsewhere. Let me tell you why.
      I went to Alma mostly because it began with the letter A. I started applying to colleges alphabetically and then, when Alma was kind enough to admit me, I lost interest in going to Zeelenopal. Who knows what would have happened if I had gone there.
      When I look back, what seems most significant is that I was safely out of my parent's hair, even though they had to pay through the teeth to keep me there. Tuition, room and board were around $2,100, and that was a lot back then.
      My parents were pleased. The unwritten code, the reason parents wanted their children to go to places like Alma, was to make this dream

come true: daughters would graduate as virgins or at least not pregnant and sons would have no discernable criminal record and would actually be sober the day of graduation. And this was the late sixties, a real accomplishment.

I tried to look academic in school, being the editor of the newspaper and yearbook. But then I was crowned Homecoming Queen, and I pretty much joined the ranks of bimbos. It was terribly embarrassing. Even then, ratting my hair to about a foot above my head, putting on the blue angora sweater and matching skirt, riding down the street on a flatbed trailer still smelling very farmish and covered with three thousand paper napkins, waving like an idiot. Even then I knew.

I have learned to deny this ever happened. If I am tortured with dental work or bamboo shoots under my nail beds, I will never admit to having been Homecoming Queen. And, once someone knows, even if I had ridden the bus with Rosa Parks or wiped the oily tears away from the dying whales, once they know, they can't seem to wipe the smirk off their faces.

So when you write for me to join the "festivities" with all the previous Queens, I wonder what you could be thinking. The way I have filled out, the graying hair and the way my elbows sort of hold up the flesh that droops from my upper arms, well, you need to put some thought into this. Who, exactly, wants to look at old bimbos?

But the real reason for this letter is to complain. I thought someone told me that a general, liberal arts degree was what I needed, what the world needed. Somehow, I thought you said there were lots of people hiring those who could talk about the Romance Period of English literature, identify an Ionic column, a sonnet, a quintet, but who didn't necessarily know how to do anything.

My first interview after college, and every one since, has never asked about any of those things. And so I went back to school to get the *real thing*. I went to nursing school at Lansing Community College where I learned a profession, a way of life really. It was inexpensive, to the point, completely bullshit-free. And they have never once called me to ask for money.

Probably no one at Alma ever counseled me wrongly. The reason for my need for a second dip was my own fault. I have very warm feelings for Alma right up to the part where I graduated and nearly fell on my face.

So please take me off your computer mailings and phone lists, and if you ever decide to get a group together to discuss the concerns and outcomes from having had the Alma experience, I am someone you can count on. I would love to be a part of a group that would help your graduates take the "right stuff" to become "the real thing."

Sincerely,

Kathleen Richards MacInnis, RN

TOUCH

I love to touch people. For some it's okay, for some, it's not. One lady was recovering from a big surgery. She had a long zipper down her belly. I told her she needed to get up and out of bed. She didn't want to, of course. I reassured her over and over and told her that I would hug her up. "Honest! It will be easy."

I held out my arms and hugged her up and out of bed. As we stood there, she tucked her head in the corner of my neck and hung on for what seemed like a long time. After a bit, I asked, "Okay?" and she slowly let go. This patient had been through major surgery and probably had been scared to death. Finally, she got what she really needed.

But other people can't be touched so easily. It takes a while for them to give permission for physical contact. Usually, they find out that being touched will not invade them, like when I first take a blood pressure. The taking of blood pressures is universal in a hospital. Sometimes I try to linger over the arm or take a pulse which, in my unit isn't really necessary. We have telemetry and can always see the heart rate. Sometimes they warm up, sometimes not. If they don't have eye contact with me, I don't look directly at them. Maybe this is like the horse whisperer. I, too, have to walk about the room, semi-disinterested in their physical selves for them to get used to me. The human whisperer.

Sometimes you can't get to know a patient if the spouse is in the room. I see a lot of sad things in my work, but these fractured, dysfunctional families are the worst. One man, it seemed, had never answered a question by himself, at least since he married the old lady. He couldn't blow his nose without being told how to use the tissues. So right away, I devised a rule that he would need brief assessments for which I was to be the only person in the room. This was needed to accurately hear lung and heart sounds.

We had some lovely visits, he and I. He seemed grateful to be able to talk, uninterrupted. Always too brief, some days he needed quite a few assessments.

WHO DECIDES THE ORDER?

Try to picture a chicken farm. Maybe one of the new ones we all hope not to ever think about where chickens are packed in, neck to neck, standing on wire grids to filter the waste, holding as still as chickens can, the farmer hoping for plump breasts and fat drumsticks. A fight breaks out and a bigger chicken begins pecking at a smaller one. Amongst the white feathers and orange brown beaks, there is arterial red blood flying. Maybe the coppery smell of blood turns the others to violence. More and more chickens join the fight, even big, strong chickens are being pecked and pecked and pecked to death. A dozen or so are lost to some unknown reason: push-come-to-shove, a just-because-I-can reason to kill another.

Things are no different at work, really. There is a pecking order for small, unseen sins. The biggest chicken begins to peck, and those who feel the sharpness of his beak or talons begin a pecking of their own on lower chickens in the order.

And on and on it goes. A housekeeper is crying in the bathroom. A new nurse thinks of quitting. A unit secretary hangs up on maintenance. It spreads like wildfire through the unit, taking innocent and guilty alike.

And then it passes and is forgotten, not because the pecking deserves forgiveness, but because there is no room to retain it all. The trash can of our relationships empties out for more memory, more peckings.

I can tell the minute I get to work if a pecking has occurred. There is something in their faces: a downcast gaze, brusque, perfunctory gestures. The landscape of a new emotional environment shows that a moat has been dug around the human psyche. We are asked not to pull down the bridge until the ego repairs itself. No eye contact, just sad looks and long sighs.

It has happened again. Someone strong has wounded someone weak. Who decides the order? What fraternity or sorority has voted on who is in, who is out? Is it our height or build, our hair color, the beauty of our facial features? What makes one person dominant over another? Education? Some invisible sign hung out for others to see that we graduated from such and so university with honors.

I know people who cannot speak without revealing where their childhood was lived: in the trailer park, a coat-hanger wire as the antenna for the most cherished piece of furniture, the TV, their mom a teenager on welfare and Medicaid with no dental care. Their words don't make them stupid, but just hint at their past.

What if you are born to privilege? Maybe you studied abroad and worked hard at your education. Nothing was handed to you, other than the constant reminder, the template given to you by your family: you must not fail, or get less than As or apply for ordinary work. Raised by an autocratic father, your achievement was assumed. You must make something of yourself, be a star, reach the top. Now, even the hint of failure in yourself or others seems like fingernails clawing on a chalkboard. Your world view cannot coexist with error. You must distance yourself from imperfection.

Those on the bottom rung of the ladder know about imperfections, they know about the pecking order. Those on top worry that failure of any kind might be contagious. By mere association, they will be seen as failures. All is driven by fear.

And so we don't look at each other. Eyes cast down if you are delivering a tray for food service, or pushing a broom. Eyes straight ahead if you are made to feel important by your pager and title and busy schedule and office staff.

We pass each other in the hall, adrift and alone. Unless something has disrupted the balance and a volley of recriminations has been made from top to bottom.

The human face plays a fascinating role in our emotional lives, telling others what our tongues do not, giving hints, sometimes dead-on accurate of the contents of our hearts. Even moments after birth, the mother reaches for her baby to look upon his face to see who this new being is. If there is bonding, if the mother cradles the child and frequently tries to look into the baby's eyes, then she has made the strong and necessary attachment that will sustain them both. Taken from the French language, this is called *en face*.

Babies only days old will track faces and seem fascinated by pictures of faces. They seem partial to faces that smile, and look away from pictures of angry people. If this is true and we are given some instinctual trait to look at faces and desire the human smile, what possible evolutionary reason could this be?

No matter how trite the words now seem, "Have a nice day!" said by checkout clerks all across America, over and over, perhaps this banal pleasantry is somehow incrementally necessary to our wellbeing. The little nudge that pushes the balance weight left or right to counteract the small slights and insults we receive each day.

I don't think we can discount the need for human kindness. Or eye contact. Or smiles.

I think we all know where we are on the chicken farm. And sooner or later, whether we deserve them or not, we will receive the dominating insults from someone else who knows he can. Sometimes even the smallest gesture of kindness, a soft word or look from one human face to another will put back the balance before we lose our footing.

FROGS

Supposedly, frogs have such basic wiring that they can't decipher hot from cold when it comes on gradually. A frog will jump right out of hot water to safety, but when placed in a pan of cold water and heated up slowly, it will stay in the pot and boil to death. I know a few people like that. Staying forever in a crumbling situation, not jumping out, unable to feel the heat.

DILATION

I walked a woman to the bathroom one day. She insisted she had to have a BM and would not consider using the commode. Against my better judgment, we got there all the same, but as I sat her down on the stool, she sort of slumped into my arms. I tried to right her, and yelled at her (this always helps) "Margaret, Margaret, are you okay?" She looked right at me, and I watched her pupils dilate, her already pale skin turn grey and wet beads form around her lips. Others came rushing in, a strip from the monitor at the desk showed asystole. A really long run of... nothing. But she somehow gained her footing, resuming a heartbeat and even woke up a little. Enough to wail that she was not finished as we carried her back to her bed for more definitive care than me yelling her name loudly.

In one culture, I think Eastern European, they believe the soul leaves through the eyes at death. And when someone is murdered, you can see the image of who did the crime, recorded on the back of the victim's eyes. I wondered if I had been recorded in the moment her eyes opened? She didn't die then. She waited until the next day.

FORE!

There are always a bunch of apocryphal stories that surround each ER and gradually seep up the stairways to the floors. The guy, in the early 80s, back when disco-dancing was so popular, that passed out from drink or drug, and once undressed was found to have about eight inches of kielbasa taped to one leg, near his groin.

The resident that was killed defibrillating a patient, leaning too close to the bed, his stethoscope touching the metal rail and becoming the conduit. These always happened HERE, at our very own hospital and were used as warnings or purely as entertainment.

One time I assisted a physician in removing a golf ball from a young woman's vagina. We all had to run through the one-liners: some foreplay... did he use a club and was this really a hole-in-one...(and of course, as it was being removed, were we to yell FORE!)

She didn't seem all that embarrassed, though we didn't draw any labs on her. I would guess the booze helped. By that time, I had given birth to two boys and wondered that something like a golf ball could get stuck in there, when the head of my ten-pounder didn't.

I also helped another physician do a vaginal exam on a 92-year-old woman who would not part with her panties, really knee-length underwear. Threading the speculum up the pant leg, making a little left turn, then trying to park it somewhere, preferably the vagina. Only to find the source of the abdominal pain: a runaway cancer. She got through it and the doctor talked at length with the family. Hospice was going to do an assessment and get her pain under control. He said later that, at the very least, she would not die prematurely, and probably would die with her panties on.

GIFTED

My son, Scott, tested well. They told me he was "gifted." I wondered if I could get a refund, like the unwanted, wrong-sized things from Christmas. Off in space most of the time, he was supposed to be with the blue birds instead of the woodpeckers. He didn't seem aware of this. How could he when his head was filled with feathers?

But messages from school never passed his lips. After dinner one night, he wanted to make pierogis, with my help. Hum. I said sure, maybe sometime, but why? And, anyway, we didn't have all the ingredients or a reliable recipe. Well, it seemed he needed enough pierogis for 23 the next day because his report on Poland was due. Poland? Due? And a costume; could he borrow a Polish costume from me?

NO BUTTS

After smoking for 50 years, my aunt died of lung cancer. But I still didn't quit. Nor did I, when, working in a hospital as a lab tech, I saw *lots* of people dying from the effects of smoking. Not even after seeing a man smoke a cigarette through his trach. But I quit when I saw my two-year-old "smoking" on the sofa one day. He had taken his Tinkertoys and was relaxing with his little short legs sticking straight out. He struck the "match": one small section and lit the Tinkertoy he had sticking in his mouth. Then he let his little shoulders rest back on the sofa and he put one arm up on the cushion while he crossed his legs, all the while taking in a deep breath. The memorized body language told me one thing. Nothing I would ever say would keep him from trying to smoke as a teenager. He's 30 now. I quit when he was two. Now, guess who smokes?

WHO'S AT THE DOOR?

In home care nursing, the bag technique is like changing your underwear without taking off your clothes. I don't miss that. In the bag, you're supposed to have the clean section and the dirty part. You are supposed to rub down equipment between uses. It's a lot of hygiene and seems to imply that the patients and their homes are extremely dirty. It always amused me, especially if these patients were to find out that I had eaten the muffin that had rolled around on the floor of my car on the way to their house. So much for clean technique.

One time I was met at the door by a woman wearing only her bra and accompanied by three cocker spaniels. Even the bra was pretty useless, being backwards, around her waist, the way some women do to fasten it before pulling it on. The three dogs were very glad to see me when they found out about the dog treats in my bag. It was a hard visit in some ways, hard to hear her lungs or heart with my stethoscope being licked. I hated throwing psych and social work her way. But answering the door that way probably wasn't a good idea.

SPOTS

Rob and I made it to the University of Michigan. We were to see the head of plastic surgery and had waited months to get the appointment. Nothing could prepare us for their waiting room. People without noses. Frankenstein-like metal cages surrounding heads and shoulders, burns that had left people with tight purple-pink skin on arms and necks and faces. You could almost see them reaching into the flames, the scars lined up on one side. And we were there just for moles. Lots of them.

For some unknown reason, Rob had been born with hundreds of moles, "giant hairy nevi." It looked almost as though he had been curled up with his butt to the front, and my swollen abdomen had been sprayed with spots. Spots that had landed on his head, back, arms and legs, but almost all on the backside. We got opinions and second opinions and then 30 opinions during grand rounds and learned that half the doctors thought we should get them off for cosmetic reasons and the other half for protection from the increased risk of melanoma. We did it for both.

It was never clear why he had them. Of course, I beat myself up lots of times wondering if I had done some terrible pre-natal thing. I told Scott, his older brother, that it was the raisin bagel I had eaten the day before he was born. But that explanation took on a life of its own as he began to want to show off his baby brother's raisins.

Once we were in the exam room, the door opened to four flapping-coated doctors, all anxious to see the "interesting" case. Each seemed to vie for position and wanted to show off his bedside manner and rapport with the smiling, eight year-old, freckled redhead. Rob didn't seem to need to relax, especially once he realized he could keep his underpants on under the gown. He began making huge breasts of his knee caps by stretching the gown over his bent legs, straining to see himself in the mirror on the wall. When asked if he would like the moles removed, he said he didn't care. But a few sentences later, he offered that the kids at school called him "the bear." One particular mole was several inches square on his leg above his sock. One of the interns asked him "how does that make you feel?" Rob told him he felt fine, but had hurt his knee the other day kicking his brother. They didn't try to psych him after that.

It seemed he could be worked into the schedule, several months from now. "Surgery is very busy; we'll have to see." But when I sat down with the office girl to fill out the forms, I learned we could be fit in at the end of next week. It seems we have insurance.

SURGERY

Rob and I made it to his surgery. He walked into the OR suite in his red bathrobe and blue flip-flops and hopped right up on the table. Basking in the attention and in awe of the spotlight and complex instruments, he said impishly, "Okay, let's get crackin' here, I haven't got all day!" Five doctors, six assistants and a little more than four hours later he was in recovery, reported to be doing fine.

Fine seemed to mean barfing the moment he awoke, and even some through the next day. (Just like his mom, his stomach seemed to hate anesthesia.) In between these little eruptions, he slept his chemical sleep. When he did awaken, his eyes were black with dilation in the darkened room, his cheeks pink with a low-grade fever. He wanted chicken nuggets. And then he was out again.

I felt like crying when it was over. Then, and every time I came or went from his four-bed room, the only room available when he came from surgery: the pediatric rehabilitation unit.

Derrick and Jonathan and Peter, beautiful children who were dying slowly from some horrible twist of fate, were his roommates. Spinal cord snapped in two, a brain crushed or tormented with relentless growing tumors.

What had Rob and I been doing that August evening when Derrick was wrestling with his friends? His neck had gone "snap" and he was forever hostage to a ventilator, his hands and feet limp and somehow just ornamental. Every morning after his bath the nurses would dress him and get him ready for his therapy. Perfect white Reebok high-tops were wedged on his lifeless feet, then positioned in the chair, just so. Never to become mud-covered or smelly like the ones my sons have scattered near our front door.

And why, on that September afternoon, had a drunken driver gone through that red light, smashing into Jonathan's family car? "Pop," had gone his brain stem, leaving him to drool and smile aimlessly at nothing. Gone was the math whiz and budding concert pianist. Though the staff did get him up each day, his feet were too misshapen to be coaxed into leather shoes. He wore instead the crocheted booties that his mother made for him.

And what if Peter hadn't told his mother on that long ago June day that he felt a little dizzy, would he now just be okay? "Mush," goes his brain each time they take him down to radiation therapy. Only to return to the room for an afternoon of helpless vomiting and drug-induced sleep.

But still they looked forward to things. One boy couldn't wait until the next day to learn to use an air straw. He wanted to play video games with his teeth.

We were there just for moles. I'd eaten right, not taken even so much as an aspirin during Rob's wonderful pregnancy. And for this I was rewarded with a noisy, beautiful baby boy with spots. Where had they come from?

I remember I had been involved in a "double code" in the ER when I was five months pregnant. A prostitute and her pimp had tried to cut each other up; both were actually dead on arrival. As we attempted to resuscitate their lifeless bodies, X-rays were taken of their blood-filled chests. During the mayhem of the moment, I didn't know they were shooting film and didn't wear a lead apron.

"Of course it wasn't from that," my doctor tried to reassure me. "Especially at five months, and the rads were so diffuse and..." He was probably right. What could I have been making at five months? Skin? Spots?

Still, we were so much better off than the other boys in Rob's room. And, as if their illnesses were not already sad enough, their families and home lives made them seem even worse. Moms that never came to visit. A dad that was ashamed of his child now that he would never play football. Fragile relations crushed with the pressure of their children's losses.

The nurses were wonderful; the doctors were excellent. But even so, I could barely leave Rob's side. I came at 6 a.m. and left only after meeting the midnight shift, 14 hours later. Because it seemed, somehow, that they were these friendly, kindly vultures with outstretched wings saying, "Go on, go get some rest. We'll watch your child for you," all the while wiping fresh egg yolk from their beaks. Of course, there was hardly anything wrong with Rob. But wasn't there a chance they could come into the nest and accidentally get the wrong egg?

We went home at week's end. The ride home was punctuated with the helium balloons his aunt sent to the hospital, floating around the back seat until they escaped accidentally at the drive-through window at McDonald's. Rob was such a trouper, no whining, really no pain, just itching now.

I guess I'm glad we did it. He looks like he went through a paper shredder with little cuts here and there and all over. He feels betrayed that no one told him he had to hold still so long. He wants to ski and sled and build snow forts. "Nobody said I had to hold still for a month!" I try to explain about the little white lies grownups tell. We knew he didn't know. But I think about how it will be when he is 18 and swimming with friends and his skin is not covered with brown hairy moles.

He has already changed the subject. I am his entertainment center. It was a mistake to buy the Wheel of Fortune game. I have had to be Vanna White all week. He doesn't get the word until almost the very last letter. He hoards his money and won't break down and buy vowels. And checkers. I don't mind losing honorably, but when he takes four of my checkers, bing, bing, bing, bing, just like that, I think maybe he's ready to go back to school.

He will need his education. He tells me now he wants to be a surgeon. And if that doesn't work out, he will go to school to be an actor. Like he already has the surgeon thing down, but he would need education to be an actor. Hmmm.

Now might be a good time to take that extra Prozac.

CURTAINS

Paul must have died around two a.m. on Christmas morning. His 42-year-old systems had kept his spinal cord cancer well supplied. His illness was short and his demise quick.

In the next bed was John, whose anger and incorrigible spirit had kept his lung cancer at bay. John and Paul had become "that room," the one no nurse wanted to find on her assignment.

John and Paul were allies in their fight against disease and somehow had come to think of us as the enemy. Nothing was sacred to them: they approached death bluntly, each betting $20 on who would "croak" first.

John was the first to know Paul had gone. His call light went on. "Someone get in here! That son of a bitch beat me. Boy, he has balls!" he bellowed. John's fists were flailing about; he looked like a commuter left behind at the train station. Grumbling, cursing, he dug through his night stand as I began to care for Paul's body, behind the pulled curtain.

"Do you want to talk?" I asked. "Talk? To you? Hell no. I want to talk to Paul. Here, put this damned thing in his hand," he said. I came around the curtain to find him handing me a $20 bill, his face defiant. "I can't do that," I pleaded, secretly wishing they had worked out arrangements for the postmortem collection of winnings. "He's dead."

"Course you can. Just put it in his hand. Do it! I don't care if the funeral director lines his pocket." I took the bill, folded it twice and put the small square in the mottled palm. From behind the curtain, I said, "Okay, he has it now."

Silence settled over the room. I was grateful. On two previous occasions, we had to close the door on this room because John and Paul were singing loud choruses of "The worms crawl in, the worms crawl out, the worms play pinochle on your snout..."

Finally, the physician appeared to pronounce Paul. Then, from behind the curtain, came John's voice: "You two gonna do something with that body before it starts to smell?"

How could I comfort this man? And even if I could, I was losing patience. It was Christmas. Paul was dead. I was here being insulted, not home with my family. But I gave it one more try.

"Are you afraid of dying, John?" I asked, inadvertently adding more fuel to the fire. "So, you're gonna sit around and talk to me with a stiff in the next bed," he raged, fueling my fire.

"No, I'm not. I am going to wait for the orderly and, together, he and I will move Paul's body out. Since you don't want to talk, I suggest you get some sleep. Your family will be here later and they'll want to spend Christmas with you."

"Don't give me that Christmas crap," he trailed off. I left the room.

Aftermath crowded the next few hours. Finally, I returned to strip the linen and raise the bed for the housekeeper to wash and remake in the morning. When I pulled the curtain back, I found John relentlessly awake. As I walked to the door, he began again. "Damn it, pull that curtain or get me a different room! That was his bed. Don't leave it up in the air with no sheets on it."

A few days later, John was having a particularly tough time breathing. He had become sullen, barely answering questions with a yes or no. I sat with him for a while. "You don't want to talk about it, so I will," I told him. "Are you worried about how it will go for you at the end?" He would not look at me, but the silence told me he was asking.

"I'll be honest with you. You'll work very hard to breathe, since it's your lungs. As it gets harder to breathe, we'll sit you up with pillows, even while you sleep. We'll give you pain medicine, but I don't think you'll have much, really. Mostly, you'll just be very tired, working for your air. When you go into a coma, the breathing will get uneven. Then it will stop. That's it, John. That's probably how it will be."

He now was looking directly at me. I wished he'd look away. After a long silence, he asked, "What if there's no coma and I'm awake and I can't breathe?"

"It seems there's always a coma," I told him. "Anyway, if you don't look like you're going to go with one, I'll use a baseball bat to knock you out."

"You will?" He smiled. "Sure," I told him. Then he began to settle down.

When I checked back with him, I said my goodbyes and without thinking added, "When your family came on Christmas, was Santa good to you?"

What followed was a lengthy berating of Christianity. Jesus wasn't going to cure him of cancer, Paul wasn't coming back, there was no life after death and he was sick of it all.

Actually, by the time he finished, he looked quite pleased with himself. With whatever traces of goodwill I had left, I sat down with him.

It seemed the gloves were off. We had finally gotten to the real stuff. I asked him about his upbringing and what he believed. "Nothin'," was his response. Then I asked him about what had been his best day, ever. And he proceeded to tell me his "best day" story.

"It's no big deal," he began. John had worked in the coal mines in West Virginia. One day, the walls collapsed and 20 men were trapped. Eighteen died from the toxic gases, but one made it out because of John. He remembered seeing the long white shaft of light above him as he helped the man out of the mine. The company awarded him a $20 bonus for his incredible bravery – a lot of money back in 1935.

This story seemed a turning point, a better way to help John. We started to share some pleasant words and eventually, when his ability to speak weakened a week later, I found even short phrases brought a smile to his eyes.

I called him "Hero," or asked about getting the baseball bat, and every time I was rewarded by a little twinkle in his eyes.

By the end of the first week in January, he had slipped badly. Seeing him struggle so hard for air, I put the over-bed stand and pillow in front of him and got his arms over it. I showed him how he could put his head down to rest. But when I went to the bathroom for a washcloth, I heard a thud. My orth-opnic lesson plan was on the floor. He was going to be a character, even to the end.

After I made my first rounds, I sat with him, silently. This, more than anything, seemed to help him. Throughout the night, I checked on him. Close to morning, I knew I might not see him again. It was close. I leaned over close to his ear and said, "You okay?" He gave me a weak nod. Then he whispered almost imperceptibly, "Merry Christmas."

I think those were his last words. It seemed like maybe a late thank-you. Probably, I was reading a lot into two little words, but that's what I heard. The next shift told me he had slipped into a coma and, not too long after that, his ragged breathing mercifully stopped.

As I got off the elevator the next night, I felt a wave of anger wash over me. There, at the end of the hall was John's bed in high position, the mattress unmade, and the curtain pulled halfway. I knew then how he had felt about Paul's empty bed on Christmas night.

I still miss John. I miss the energy I'd seen him use to rail at death. I miss his ability to believe in not believing. And if he was ill-behaved and difficult, that made it all the sweeter when I could get a brief glimpse at his awkward attempts at kindness. I'll always believe he was saying, "Thank you," when he said "Merry Christmas."

IN MY POCKET

As I stuff the washer with my three days of uniforms, I pull from the pockets the four-fold papers I use for report. Room number, name, age, doctor and all the history in an alphabet soup of abbreviations for the illnesses that plague a person past his prime: GERD, HTN, CAD, CHF, BPH, low EF. This guy is pretty good, just waiting for an AICD, an implanted device to give his heart a shock if it goes into a very bad rhythm. Then, home tomorrow.

All is routine until I find the folded paper from the day I floated to the ICU. Both sides covered with the lengthy reports, one man, quite stable, waiting to be flown out to another hospital to have a specialized procedure done on his aneurysm. Another, 19 years old, in a coma after flying through the air from his snowmobile and hitting a tree. His mother is focused on the eyelid that doesn't work. "When will he be able to open his left eye?" she keeps asking. To see what? A blown pupil, no real response, and when he postures, she believes he's pushing us away intentionally.

Both are heads. I hate heads. The big computer of the body, the window to the soul. The repository of all that makes us human; the cells that tell us song and smell and sight and every other sensation. And memory, the enormous card catalogue that instantly flips to our past: this is a face I know, this is how to put my shoes on, that is the perfume my daughter wears.

And it seems always the loved ones of the heads are the toughest of them all: distraught, angry, vigilant. They seem to do their homework in double time, knowing about any and all case reviews on the Internet. It seems always to fall to the nurses. The families are relatively pleasant with the physician but, when he leaves, they turn their frustrations to the ones at the bedside.

The washer is churning in full cycle. I toss the papers away. I'll have clean uniforms and new sheets of paper to fill. But my patients' stories stain my head. No washing can get them out, except by dilution from more folded papers.

INAPPROPRIATE

I don't often talk about my mom. In my life, she has been dead more years than I have been alive, dying at 64 when I was just 30, a sudden big bleed the size of a peach in her head.

She lived about a day and a half after her stroke. My sisters and I rushed to the ER after frantic calls. She had been so full of life, packing to go on a trip to Pennsylvania to see her ailing sister.

When I saw her in the ER, she was comatose. Maybe she squeezed my hand. I thought so then. I just lost it. I became belligerent with the physician who tried to tell us how bad the prognosis was. I grabbed him by the lapels, and pulled him close to my face and said in a low, even growl, "What do you mean she will die? Who do you think you are?"

I stopped. I was deeply embarrassed. I slid back to a corner of the room and began sobbing. Those awful gasps, trying to not make noise, when the air escapes and you begin to blubber and snot pours out of your nose.

He stayed with us and didn't call security. He waited and then said to all of us, "It's okay, I know this is hard."

Mom and I had our differences. She would take me under her wing but it seemed more like a headlock. She loved me, but her affections were surrounded by a moat filled with alligators. So, we kept the drawbridge up. It was better for both of us that way.

At her funeral, I met people with so many kind things to say about her that I wasn't sure I was at the right service. Who was this woman? I loved her as my mom. I would never know her has a woman, teenager, sister, or dear and loyal friend. By the time I knew her and dad, they were already corrupted by children – us.

I acted out one more time. When they were preparing to put her in the ground, we were supposed to leave the cemetery, not stay to watch. I kept thinking I didn't want that guy to touch her box. He was huge and his pants were low enough to see his crack in back and his belly button in the front, with lots of hair. Big sweat rings under each arm, his shirt torn, almost no teeth, chewing on a wad.

I pulled away from the group that was walking back to the car and waited, thinking I would supervise her interment. But worse than having this man be the last person to touch her wooden box of ashes, his assistant in the distance was driving a backhoe over the lawn toward us. Someone pulled on my arm, made me get in the car and we drove away.

She might not have been easy in life. But it seemed I could easily rip apart with my teeth anyone who messed with her in death.

I think, somehow, she might have liked my outbursts on her behalf. Though of course, she would have told me I had been "inappropriate."

INVISIBLE LINKS

With one strong cramp, the baby slipped out between my legs. At only two month's gestation, it didn't look human – the gnarled gray rubbery thing couldn't have been a real baby to anyone else. But to me it was the child I was supposed to have.

I thought to call her Ann. I made a nest of Kleenex for her. As I held this two-inch twist of tissue, the "products of conception," as my doctor called it, the paper blankets began to soak with moisture, making a halo of pale cherry around her gray body. I placed her gently on the floor. After drying myself off, I went to the kitchen to get a plastic bag. I slid her in it, put it on top of the half-full wastebasket, and carefully covered it with clean dry tissues.

It was two days before I emptied the basket. I went into the hospital that night for a D and C. The next day I mostly rested on the couch. When I walked in the bathroom I would circle the basket, checking to see that the tissue layer was undisturbed, pacing around it as if caught in some circumference that held me there. And then it didn't anymore. I took out the trash. And got on with my life.

After my mom died, I went to the house to dismantle her belongings, to set in motion once again a household that had been filled with activity until the last moment when sudden death robbed her of old age. I removed the bed linens carefully, thinking that something of her was still in those pieces of cloth.

She had dry skin, I reasoned. Wouldn't at least one cell of my mother still be left, cast off from her elbow or heel?

A day later, I returned to find my thoughtful husband had washed everything: the blankets, spread and the precious wrinkled sheets with something of my mom still in them.

I thought I might be the only one, the only crazy person. But about a month after my dad died, my sister sent me an old sweater of his in a plastic bag with a note attached: "Smell this! Doesn't it smell just like him?"

My friend Barb recently learned that her mother has been sleeping with her dead husband's leg bag for more than a year. Her mom wasn't home, so Barb thought she'd help by making the bed while waiting for her return. There it was in the bed. Her father had died after a long slow struggle with cancer. Barb's mother had cared for him up until the end, turning him, bathing him, giving him the morphine, and emptying his catheter bag.

As Barb told me about her mother, her eyes filled with tears. Her own loss mixing with the fears for he mother's mental health confused her. She said she'd talked to her mom, but her mom just got mad. "She exploded! I couldn't believe it. She said she wasn't ready yet."

When I was little, I used to daydream about putting a message in a bottle and launching it in the ocean. It would float to England or France and someone would find it. And the paper inside would have been touched by me and then by their hands. It seems we are connected by invisible small links, like a note in a bottle, touching each other in some way.

My baby girl, my mom's dry skin, the smell of my father... I understand about the leg bag. It seems these things connect us in some way. They make some kind of bridge until we can let go.

I know what Barb's mother felt. I think I know what it feels like when you're not ready to let go, and then, for reasons I can't explain, you are.

JUMPING THE CURB

For some time, I have been giving talks to groups about my work as a nurse for Hospice. I'm good at it. I love being a nurse and I love to talk. But the telling of my Hospice work means I must accept the risks that come with telling.

The audience reaction to my remarks is predictable. I say the words they hope I won't: death, dying, terminal. I even do a fairly detailed commentary on bowel movements, though never at a luncheon. My listeners will be interested or afraid. With some, we have eye contact, and I can bet they are going to ask questions, even interrupt with stories of their own. Quite often, they have had a death happen in their family and when it was a positive experience, they can't wait to say so.

Others are playing with a paper clip, doodling, crossing their legs back and forth, scratching, sleeping. But nothing will make them look at me. It's like I'm not even there. They may have come from families that can't talk easily about a lot of things or, maybe, they have had a bad experience with a death.

I usually tell them how I had done all kinds of nursing and was getting tired of the ICU thing with too much intervention on the very old or very sick and how it seemed inhumane to poke and prod someone who faces overwhelming odds. So I left the hospital setting and began driving to the homes of people who had chosen to become our Hospice patients.

I always tell them how happy the patients are to not have uncomfortable tests, chemo or radiation therapy. Some even get "better," like going on a honeymoon for a while and their symptoms seem almost to go away. I tell about the morphine or other drugs for pain, and how we try to prevent nausea and restlessness and depression. About how we pay for a lot of stuff, because of our reimbursement process, though there is never enough money to go around. But the families do not have to pay for us to be there and for some families, signing on with Hospice is a big financial relief.

We send to the home a nurse and an aide, a social worker who can help sort through the tangles of issues that come up near the time of death. We always offer, but never push a spiritual advisor or we make contact with their own faith if they wish. Our volunteers befriend and sit with the patients when their loved ones have to be away. And we offer post-care of support groups and counseling, even for very young children.

I talk about how we're all going to die and I think of myself as a "midwife of death" because I have seen it so many times and know the signs and symptoms of approaching death. I can help explain, comfort and reassure them as they go through the stages.

And then I tell them about Joe. He was, by far, my favorite patient and I never know how I will make it through the telling. It's different every time. He had lung cancer and smoked to the very end. His family and wife were supportive and he even had a great dog, though she worried me a lot the night he died. When the funeral home guys came for the body, she was holding a vigil under the hospital bed and her low growl seemed sadly ominous.

There are so many stories about Joe that I have to think about which ones to include. The time he nearly burned the house down? The pack of Marlboros the family put me up to sneaking into the casket so the priest wouldn't see them doing it? The time we all cheered when I delivered a much needed BM?

In today's talk, I told about the nightgown. I'd been talking for most of 30 minutes. It was like driving down a road in a familiar neighborhood, making Joe come alive again for my audience. Driving, maybe a little too fast, but still, knowing all the turns.

Overnight, Joe had been incontinent and had messed up his last clean hospital gown. That morning, I arrived to find Joe in a light blue nightgown, all cleaned up but a nightie all the same.

Because we were good friends and had long ago lost any pretense of formality, I began my stand-up comedy routine about how you never know someone until they are out of the closet.

Then I stopped. Something made me stop. Joe said it was his mom's nightgown, from when she had been so sick. It had Velcro closings at the back. And he really liked wearing it; it made her feel close. In fact, he thought he'd seen her, clear as day, last night standing at the end of his bed. Just smiling at him.

I couldn't go on. My throat made little wet clicking sounds. There was one dry sob that escaped. My tire went over the curb. I took a breath. I waited. Now everyone was looking at me, even the guy who'd been asleep in the corner.

I waited, holding the back of a chair with both hands. And then I closed. I told them Joe was making his transition. From that time on, he began to die in earnest, after seeing his Mom. Almost as though he was looking forward to it.

I told them I love this work, even if it makes me cry sometimes. It's because of the people like Joe, that I do it.

All four tires got back on the pavement. There were a few questions. Some people started to leave, go for a smoke or whatever. One or two came up to thank me. Their eyes were a little red.

I think that Joe was a remarkable patient, living on and on. It's good to tell this story, so maybe more patients can have a good death. And I'm glad I took the risk to tell it.

MAKING GOODBYES

Dear Dying Person,

As a nurse, I have seen a lot of people die. And, though each death was sad, some were better than others. Expectant couples take classes to prepare for the birth of their child. I think someone should talk with you about preparing for death. There *is* such a thing as a good death. But it may mean you have to talk about the things your family and friends are trying to avoid. So here goes.

1. Get a confessor. Early on, find someone with whom you can talk "dirty." A friend, nurse, physician, or family member who will allow you to say words like dead, kick the bucket, croak, tumor, cancer. All those things you and your loved ones are thinking about but are too polite to say out loud. Say them. It won't hurt and you'll feel better.

2. You have as many rights as you did a year ago or 10 years ago. You need not spend the days or weeks or months ahead in pain or depression or anxiety. Don't let someone convince you that you'll become addicted to narcotics or that your depression would lift if only you had a better spiritual life. You may not have quantity left but you can demand the best quality. Insist on good pain control. And with the chemical changes of your disease at work, maybe you could benefit from medicines for depression or anxiety.

3. You're not dead yet. So don't act like it any more than you have to. My friend's son was hospitalized with leukemia at St. Jude's Hospital for Children. There, as long as they can, the children make their beds and put the toys back on the shelf. One child made his own bed until the day before he

died. It helps you and those who love you when you do what you can.

4. Have you decided what to wear at your funeral? Honoring your wishes will comfort your family after death. You may even take some satisfaction in knowing that your desire for cremation or burial will be fulfilled.

5. Have you ever read about or talked with anyone who has had a near-death experience? Possibly your nurses have heard stories from their patients. Ask them. Scientific proof and religious backgrounds aside, please think about this with an open mind. Not enough nice things are said about death; it gets a lot of bad press. The patients I have talked to really enjoyed being dead and didn't want to come back. Maybe you'll like it.

6. Everybody dies. There's nothing to be ashamed of. Joggers die. Health-food advocates die, and so do people who have spent their entire lives in a La-Z-Boy recliner eating corn curls and drinking Miller beer. Don't muddy it all up feeling guilty. If you've been told you're going to die soon, the only word that should bother you is "soon."

7. Do you have some deep dark worry that you find hard to confess? I don't mean the real story about Aunt Marion's diamond ring or that little thousand-dollar dent in the Ford. I mean the nitty-gritty; the mechanics of death. Maybe your confessor can help you with this. Stuff like, what happens when you stop breathing? Or your heart stops? Will you feel it? Are you worried that you'll look or smell terrible? I worry that my handsome prince will lean over my bed to kiss the lips of his Sleeping Beauty and I'll have dog breath. I probably will. But even saying this to someone seems to help.

8. Do you want music at your last moments? A special reading, or candles burning? Who should be there? I'd like to have my husband. My sons, too, although their attention span was pretty short when they were teenagers and they probably would get bored. The ones I really want are my dog and cat, though the cat will only come if it's convenient for her.

9. Consider having a "living" wake. This might help with unfinished business, to say some goodbyes or express regrets or thanks but, more important, it would celebrate

your life. Everyone invited would be asked to bring a story of times they had fun with you, or learned from you, or they shared in your life. It would be a time to care for those who are close to you. Maybe old movies, photos, Bible readings. I love the part where Jesus is nearing the end, and he tells his disciples, "take care of my mother...watch over one another..." You may also want to contribute in some way.

I certainly don't know all the answers. These are just suggestions. But among the dying patients I have cared for one questions recurs: "Can we talk?" Talking about death is as difficult as talking about sex. But when I have talked "dirty" with my patients, when they have whispered their deepest fears and concerns, they seemed to gain a measure of peace. Always, I learned more than I taught. I felt honored to be their listening friend. Don't hold back; get some help. Then give it your best shot. You probably will only get one chance to die. In the end. you'll have to do it alone. Make the byes good.

THE MORGUE IS COLD

I never really minded taking people to the morgue. To me it's the last thing I can offer and I'm at least doing something, not standing around wringing my hands.

One hospital where I worked used shrouds. I had a terrible time folding the white plastic sheet over the face. After all, it is the very thing every mother dreads. I would think, "What if the patient tries to breathe?" (I was also the child who would become hysterical if my dolls were put in a bag and loaded in the trunk with the rest of the luggage. How could they breathe?)

One time, I had to take a lady to the morgue to meet up with her leg. Her leg had been amputated and was carefully wrapped and waiting for her in a drawer in the cooler. I guess a body part that big is given special treatment. At any rate, it had pre-deceased her by a week.

I never could get used to one supervisor on nights who insisted that *no* cover be put on the body before being placed in the cooler. She explained that the point of the cooler was to preserve the body and my good idea of two flannel blankets would be counterproductive. But graves often have blankets: those tacky fake grass ones. I also wondered about leaving a small light on, like those book clip-on lights. It was pretty dark in there. That suggestion didn't go anywhere, either.

When I was young, my sister and I helped conduct about a dozen pet funerals in our backyard. We saved shoe boxes just for this purpose. Birds, one beheaded frog, cats. Dogs were more than we could handle. Mostly we specialized in the under-served strays or homeless dead, who fertilized a space behind our garden. We used a prayer book, and set up small chairs for our bereaved friends who would only learn of the dead at the funerals. They looked appropriately saddened all the same.

MARY THE WELSH CORGI DOG MACINNIS

Mary went quietly to sleep last week, in our arms. By the time we had taken her to the veterinarian, it was the only thing to do. I will miss her terribly. She will be my Christmas tree dog. Just as you can find needles behind the couch even in July, I am still finding her hair everywhere. A broken dog biscuit in the car, the calendar of Corgis doing all the cute things they do. I will miss her most because she made me laugh. It was like living with happiness every day.

I went to the Hallmark store to see about some cards to send. But I only found angel dogs with birds. I guess Mary did like the dead birds she found by the side of the road – something to roll in. But then I thought about religious cards, that maybe I could draw some dogs as the disciples, each wearing a Middle Eastern bathrobe and sandals, sitting on its hind legs, arms propped on the table. There'd be a little elbowing, some good natured growling. But still they would share the Purina chow and water in the saucer passed between them.

Then the problem arose of who would be Jesus. What species could lead the pack, so to speak? A big yellow Lab with soft brown eyes? A Collie taken from America's long love affair of Lassie, coming straight from the small black and white TV screens of the 1950s? But what if this card had come from the East? Wouldn't it necessarily have 12 little kimono-clad Shar-Peis? Probably that's why no one has attempted to make a line of religious dog cards.

I wish I could thank my distant relative, the caveman who first tossed a bone over his shoulder, to be appreciated by the wolf that was drawn to the light of the family fire. I sometimes wonder if the wolf-dog would have come back the next night if he could have foreseen his future of grooming with little bows on each ear, or shock collars to remind him to stay in the yard. Or the long waits for his owners to return or the hopelessly inadequate walks and attention.

I don't know. I have regrets but, somehow, it seemed Mary had a bad memory. She never held a grudge. She always seemed to admire everything I did. No matter what my intellect told me, I always saw a little of Jesus in the eyes of my dog. The dog I have to give back to God. That's just it. Everything has to go back. Everyone we love is only on loan. Even if only for a few short years, how wonderful we get them at all.

THE RAIL

I had a dream last night, so clear, so terrifyingly real that I awoke with tears pouring from my eyes, my throat tight with fear. It was a dream of my father, who has been lost to disease and afflictions for many years. Yet he is like some toy boxing clown that pops back up relentlessly after every punch, and never goes down for the count. He has Alzheimer's disease. And it seems he is in a battle for what is left of his brain.

I dreamed I went to his apartment. It was an October evening. I remember it was dusk. The door was ajar and the rooms dark. I was instantly angry with my mother to think she had gone out without dad when I had called to arrange the visit. (Mom's been dead seven years and dad lives in a nursing home.)

I wandered through the rooms, one after another, but all the while I heard the low moan of what I thought must be an injured animal. I found dad out on the small deck, standing near the rail. Where was mom? Why was he alone, I wondered? It was past eight and nearly dark, just shadows now in the cool almost cold night air. Here he was in his boxer shorts and shirt stained with food and only one button in place. Over and over, he moaned.

"Dad," I said, "I'm here!" "It's Katie!" But the murmuring continued. He shifted his weight backward to his heals at the sound of my voice.

His shrunken form tilted more and more until it seemed he would fall against the glass door-wall. I reached out to help him. As my hand made contact with his back, each finger, the palm and thumb were planted so firmly it seemed I had somehow slapped him. Instead of breaking his fall, it seemed that I was pushing him forward, nearer to the rail. And then over it.

He would not be sick anymore. He would not drool and urinate on the sofa; or wander out into the parking lot, opening, closing, opening, closing, over and over, other people's car doors. Mom would be free of him and, in a short time, people would forget his disease and remember only his many vital years of service and dedication as a father, neighbor and businessman. It would be a good memory of Dad; he would want it this way.

But in the time it takes for thoughts – how long, how long – he circled toward me, away from the rail and wrapped his arms around me. "Oh Frannie, Oh Frannie!" he cried, mistaking me for Mom. "I don't want to die, don't let me die... not now, not me..." he sobbed over and over, chanting, begging for his life.

I could not tell, in this black moment of my dream, the origin of his request. Was it fear of falling? Was this one lucid moment, surfacing long enough to be aware of how steadily his disease was already taking him, neuron by neuron? Or did he feel in the pressure of my hand that I not only righted him from a backward fall, but thought to push him over the rail and let him fall to the ground from the second floor?

Could he see the strobe light of the ambulance that surely would be called? Would his crumpled figure take one last breath before it was, at long last, still?

Instead, he was here in my arms. His head tucked at my neck, like a small child's, sobbing, shaking with cold and fear and age.

But then it seemed I was in his arms. Could this be the small waiting room outside the dentist's office years ago? Wasn't it my voice that I heard begging in between the moans, "No, no please!" And didn't he hold me close then? Wasn't it his hand at my back teaching me to ride the two-wheeler? And wasn't it I who came to him in early years, half-dressed, disheveled, so he could pull on and put to right some dress or coat or hat?

In my dream, I took his hand and slowly we walked back across the patio door's edge into the dark apartment. He sat, shaking on the edge of the bed as I began to draw a warm bath for him. Sometime between this good intention and accomplishment, I awoke.

The dream is gone, but the fear remains. No bath will wash away my father's disease. His real comfort will come some day in the cold embrace of death. A final knock-down, drag-out punch. But never from my hand. As I wipe the tears away from my face, I know these are not the hands that will take a life.

Years ago, so long it seems to me a dream, I was small and needed him to take my hand and lead me out of danger. My life was stretched out before me then. Dad's long life, so filled with accomplishments is behind him now. I must remember this backwards hope each time I lead him from the rail.

OUTSIDE IN THE COLD

When my Aunt Dorothy died, my dad and sister and I drove seven hours in a day just to go to the service. It was worth it. Actually, it was incredible.

Her beautiful wooden coffin was already there, near the altar, when we arrived. Resting between six tall floor candles at the end of a long aisle, so long you could hardly see the end, in this cavernous cathedral in the old-money town of Pittsburgh. A town of hard steel and ugly smoke stacks. But some steel barons became enormously wealthy, as I could easily see from the "in memory of" plaques that lined the edges of the dark walls on both sides.

Three ministers, all with deep dramatic voices, spoke the words of the service. It was a November day with a steady rain pouring down outside in the cold gray. The church interior was dark or nearly so; pillars covered with ornate wood carvings cast black shadows on the barely visible side hallways leading to still other chapels and altars and even darker corners. The windows seemed to be black tapestry, with no sun to illuminate their stained-glass saints.

The ministers read poems: "Stopping by Woods on a Snowy Evening," was one.

My uncle sobbed. Silently at first and then a small air leak escaped his clenched jaw and he whimpered like a wounded animal, not a human sound. His life had been immaculate. He was a partner of a respected architecture firm. He always dined with his coat on and used proper crystal and silver flatware. But this day his hair was long over his limp collar and his coat was lightly dusted with dandruff. His head stooped forward with the posture of his early Parkinson's disease.

My lungs hurt with the pain of muffled tears trying for control. But I lost composure entirely when, at the end, Aunt Dorothy's coffin was walked out. Silently rolling by us, with the ministers in unison chanting, "Ashes to ashes, dust to dust..." Slowly reaching the very back of the church, until the words were lost, and the last sound was the closing of the door.

Like a child who must know, literally *know* the answer, I whispered to my sister, "Where did they take her?"

"Outside, to the hearse," she answered.

The funeral guests filed out silently to the parish hall to solemnly greet the family. There, we were served a lunch of cheese soufflé and black cherry Jell-O. I will never think of black cherry

Jell-O without thinking of my Aunt Dorothy, her beautiful funeral, and her waiting for us outside, in the cold November rain, for one last ride.

SEVEN FEET TALL

Dad slipped into a coma last Sunday night; early Wednesday morning he died, more peacefully than most. At the end, it was a collapsed lung and intractable temperature, heart failure and maybe dehydration. He had not been awake for more than two weeks but, living 220 miles away, I had not known this until one of the last urgent phone calls on Sunday. At least I got to see him. Rob, my seven-year-old, and I drove down and arrived at 11 p.m. He died at 12:30 a.m. Something for a child to see. Something for a 40-year-old to see, who must try to start acting like a grownup, parentless.

He was one class act. Schooled out east, at places with names like Shady Side Academy and Lehigh University, he knew which fork to use and how to wear a tux. But he didn't like to do either. He did the husband thing and dad thing and was responsible. He was on the school board and many boards of directors. He went to work each day without fail as an industrial engineer.

One spring day, I got pneumonia and he entertained me with stories. It was then I learned from him all I know about poker. He had worked before college in the coal mines and one summer as a medic with longshoremen. He was a big man with a handshake that almost hurt and fine blue eyes that looked right at you. He swam against Johnny Weissmuller to place for the Olympics, but couldn't go on to the finals because he broke his collarbone in a fight. He told me he had broken up a fight and hit the guy square on the jaw and killed him. It wasn't considered a crime, just a thing that happened.

I always thought he could do anything. I thought he was seven feet tall. He knew how to swear so it sounded like music. He loved rare roast beef in big slabs that dripped over the plate's edge. And halfway through dinner he would order another round of drinks and light up another Marlboro, food still waiting at his place. It seemed the height of luxury to let your food grow cold, like you are the king.

When I saw him last, he weighed about 130 pounds. You could have put the bowl of a spoon in the sunken hollow beside his thumb. He was hot and working hard to breathe. And then he just sort of stopped and then began again and then stopped again. Like a fish, flip-flopping in one last agonal attempt.

It took Rob about six minutes to recover enough to begin wondering out loud which restaurants would be open at 1 a.m. That's probably a record. Even so, it was good to have him there and I learned a lot from my own lips as I began to explain why it was okay that we were going to burn Granddad's body in an oven. The part about the soul, and the body we see is just the holding place and, well, you probably know the rest. I'm still not sure about some of it, but I made a pretty convincing argument. It had been Dad's wish.

If I had *my* wish, we would be transported back to the kitchen table in our first house. Dad would be reading the morning newspaper; the date at the top would be 1955. Mom would be alive and we would all be having breakfast together as a family. The smell of coffee, the eggs and bacon. Toast popping up a little burned.

And, as we each left for school or the office or the store, we would give each other kisses on the cheek, and wish each other a good day.

It was always a good day with my dad.

WHERE THERE IS HOPE

When the biopsies and blood work confirm wide-spread metastatic cancer, when there are "doll's eyes" or tombstones on the EKG, when the lungs are stiff with years of smoking, where is hope?

To tell my patient the truth means I must tell him he will die. Of course he will, no matter what, even if I tell him nothing.

But isn't there some lifejacket I can wrap around his shoulders to encourage him? Isn't there some small thing I can suggest about therapies or medications, about diets and attitudes that somehow challenge the statistics? When I look at his chart I see the Latin words that translate: too soon, not long, not forever.

These patients seem stunned. Like a deer paralyzed by the shining headlights of a car on a country road. The animal can run to safety only when the lights go by and he is released from the spell. In the safety of the dark woods he will go on living. But another time, in another way, this animal will die.

When I talk to the very ill or dying patient, I try to think of ways to slow time. When you are first born, your parents think a week is a long time. When you have only weeks to live, there is a force, like water circling the drain, that makes a day seem only a minute long.

As a nurse, I see how important it is that this time be free of symptoms like pain and nausea. The rest is mostly up to the patient and his family. I admit to occasionally being the matchmaker, getting family members to drop their grudges and rally at the bed-side and to talk to each other. It doesn't always work.

I answer all questions. I try to tell the truth. When the patient asks what was found during surgery or if he is going to die, I try to remember one thing: do what's right. Forget the "don't talk" rule. If the doctor should have told them, I call him, even at home, and tell him they are asking.

So what if the doctor yells (as if this would be the first time!). If the results are good, I tell. If they are bad or uncertain, and it is after 11 p.m., and I can see the patient needs something, I tell him something. Always true, but maybe only part.

It helps if you ask the patient for her story. "I had these headaches right after we moved and didn't think too much about them because we had just painted a lot of the bedrooms..." "With all the coffee I drink, I had come to expect lumps in my breasts..."

They almost always want to talk. Story after story. Beginnings of what may be endings. I try to point out that, before they knew it was a tumor with a name, they were living their lives, going places, doing things. And though we now know it is something bad, they must not waste even a minute of the time left.

It is their choice, no matter what the statistics say. They can decide to fill today with as much as they did a year ago, or two years ago. And ultimately, they will decide when to die.

Occasionally, I meet an old person who seems to have mastered the heavy burdens of age. Like my patient Hilda who was very near death but continued to work her embroidery with utmost precision, pulling out and correcting the wrong stitches. She had survived the death camps in Germany during World War II, when she watched her whole family die. She had married twice, buried twice; even two children had been lost. But her days were not filled with remorse or loss so much as asking about my children and did I like rice pudding? We agreed this was one of life's pleasures.

You can say Hilda was old. Of course, she was ready for her death in a way others are not. But I have seen the same essence, the same will to stay in the now and live the now for all it's worth in an 11-year-old cystic fibrosis patient. It took one entire morning to curl her hair just right so she could be ready when the phone rang. Arrangements had been made for the lead singer of the 'New Kids on the Block' to call her in her room, "all the way from California." She looked beautiful. She was thrilled and as alive as anyone I know. Several months later, on her next admission, she died. But still, I don't remember her disease nearly as well as the twinkle in her eyes when the phone rang.

Staying well is an inside job, it seems. A place where disease does not go and chemotherapy can't reach. Essence can't be ordered up from central supply; it is not ours to give our patients.

If the deer can cross the road when my lights turn away, patients can live each day of their lives, even the last ones with hope. Giving hope to a patient is to tell her that we can see something wonderfully alive in her, even when she cannot.

DARK SUNNY DAY

This past week we have been deluged with trauma victims. Cars that crashed, off-road three-wheelers that were meant only for fun, motorcycles, everything that moves. And the people who were driving, never move again. The first night we got a young man, age 19 or so, who shot himself in the face attempting suicide. Then the next day, a man, 24, who had too many beers and no seat belt. He came to us as John Doe – brain dead. The orders said: "Support until identified, then request organ harvest from the family."

He was beautiful, tanned, his injury hardly showed and he still smelled of after-shave. He wore a gold chain and purple nylon bikini briefs which we cut off. The other boy lived about three days. Most of his face was gone, destroyed by the blast. The surgeons sewed enough together to try to stop the bleeding and performed a tracheotomy so he could breathe. His room smelled of old blood, no matter what we did. The beige, mummy-like dressing needed constant redressing since the bleeding never really stopped. Nurse after nurse was seen leaving the room with shoulders that fell oddly downward and faces stiff with fixed expressions. Going to break could not help. They did not even come down for lunch; their throats filled with the cotton of trying not to cry.

At least, at the very least, the accident victim did become a donor. Five people late that night heard their telephones ring and were asked to prepare themselves for what they prayed for and feared most. Teams of doctors came by helicopter and small planes to take away the good from the bad. His heart, kidneys, eyes and liver all in small picnic coolers with dry ice. Coolers with snappy names like "Fun Pack" and "Little Oscar."

These dramas played against a backdrop of a string of wonderfully sunny summer days. Why couldn't it be a raging winter storm? But instead, my husband and I were invited to a party with food and drink and swimming for the kids. It should have been a great relief, but it was as though my body was invited but my brain couldn't come. I searched my thoughts: what could I say that would be appropriate? The kids? My fascinating dentist appointment last week? The new tires I bought for the Ford?

Then I saw a nurse across the way. Not from my unit, but I knew her well enough to go to her and say, "how are you, our unit's been crazy, how about yours?" I never mentioned the two young men. But it was a comfort to be close to her, somehow. If I needed to be nursed, she was there. I knew that, sometime, she also had shared in the dark secrets only we knew. The forbidden knowledge only we have, it seems.

Now might be a good time to get some cheese and crackers to go with the whine.

LATE BLOOMERS

Résumés are too much like obituaries. First, they are inflexible. What's past is past and will not change any time soon. When you write down your story it can look boring or insignificant. But with résumés, you can add an addendum, right up to the end.

As I turn to "Page Two," as Paul Harvey would say, what has gone before seems insignificant. I was a crossing guard in grade school, I am a life member of Weight Watchers, and a survivor of a head injury.* These are not the things you find on résumés. And none of them resulted in the addition of letters after my name, like my learned friends can boast. I am a BARN, with a BA in liberal arts and an RN. Supposedly, you are to keep them in the order they were received.

Maybe I'll become a late bloomer. Either that, or an embarrassing, unaccomplished shallow person who only went to work, did groceries and cooking and cleaning and sewing and car pooling and volunteered at church, mowed the lawn and gardened while having children. You know the drill.

When I no longer have the excuse of "I work full time" to hide behind, when my children are themselves wrinkled and bald, then I will have to show others what a great success I am.

I look at some of the leaders in this: Grandma Moses didn't start painting until she was nearly 80. Winston Churchill was in his 70s when he led Great Britain through World War II. At 65, Groucho Marx started a brand-new career on television.

Maybe I'll become the George Plimpton of the aging baby-boomers and sample careers temporarily, checking out new options for the semi-halt, the slightly lame, and then report back. I would have a checklist of aging issues: Does this career have stairs to climb, lots of leg work or heavy lifting? What about needing to be flexible? Do I have to remain open-minded in the presence of rabid left- or right-wing people? Would I work with others my own age or be "embedded" (similar to "deep-sixed") with people who could be my grandchildren? If there were a senior discount, and free items were given to employees, wouldn't they have to pay me each time I used their product? There seems a dearth of research here.

One book suggests developing hobbies that were favorites during younger years. One man loved find wines and began his own small winery after retiring. Of course, this was in his basement, garage and guest bedroom, and a divorce soon followed. A woman began a pet-sitting business and lovingly cared for stray cats in her home until she was closed down after Animal Control found 200 dead cats in plastic bags in her backyard.

Not all of our early "tendencies" are things we should nurture as we age.

One of my great fears going into retirement is of just becoming a consumer, not a bloomer. I don't want to just shop or spend money. I don't want my life to be defined by entertainment, travel and restaurants. I don't want to be the American that goes to Chartres Cathedral in France and remembers to complain about the toilet paper in the public bathroom. Or upon returning from my travels, be able to list the restaurants that give immediate coffee refills.

I want to *do* something each day, something that actually needs *doing*. That's the kind of late bloomer I want to be! Picked for the team, up early each morning, ready to get to work, even if the job description sounds like the work of a dandelion!

* I raised two sons, both of whom had attention deficit disorder. In constant motion every waking moment, they would, miraculously, hold perfectly still watching Dukes of Hazzard. It was amazing. Like they were in a trance. I read somewhere that good parents don't just park their children in front of the TV, they sit down and watch with the child. So I did. Watching Dukes was how I got the brain damage.

OLD

I am wondering when I will be so outdated, so slow of mind and body that I will be asked to leave my job. How soon will my 24 years of nursing count for less than the young grads' bright-and-shining up-to-date education?

Will there even be time to post a note about my leaving on the staff bathroom door, enough time to have a punch-and-cookie goodbye party between hurried forays down the hall to answer call lights?

I feel like a melting candle, the light about to go out. I am no longer the strong young woman in her early 30s, fresh from nursing school, anxious for codes and procedures and every kind of new and scary thing. I couldn't wait to get to work. I loved being a nurse. I loved working in a room filled with tubes and vents and machines and monitors—and patients, too.

Now, I run the other way. Now, I'm just a big chicken. I find ways out; I talk about hair color with the wife and get coffee for the visitors. I hand out comfort meds as though I'm offering a box of chocolates to my dinner guests: something to please them, to help them forget, not feel, not remember the pain.

Why must I know what I know? Why do I continue to work on a floor of post-open hearts? Why, when the code is called and a patient is found lying diagonally on the bed, must his chest be invaded yet again? I hand the surgeon the instruments to crack open the chest of this newly dead, recently bypassed patient. The doctor tries to squeeze life back into the dark red muscle that is quivering hopelessly in the cavern of his chest. The patient's feet and hands are gray, his chest now black with blood.

A few minutes earlier, this man was in his robe and slippers walking back from the elevator where he said goodbye to his wife. His glasses are on the bedside stand, resting on a half-finished crossword puzzle.

I feel dizzy and resort to an old trick I learned as a new grad, throwing my pen to the floor. I lean over to pick it up, refilling my brain with blood.

I don't even stay to see how this story ends. I am gone when the family arrives, when the surgeon talks to them in hushed tones. I will be in the parking lot, digging in the dark for my keys when the wife is kissing the waxy cold lips of her husband for the last time.

"It's okay," I think I'd tell her. Better dead than bringing him back to life. Life in rehab for weeks or months: "This is your wife, Gladys. Can you say Glad-iss?" He was down too long, too many minutes without oxygen.

Will they sew him up, crudely, like the bulging end of a Thanksgiving turkey filled with dressing? Will he be in a box somewhere, dressed in clothes he never wore except to other people's funerals?

I don't know. I don't even want to know anymore. I have lost my edge. A drug rep arrives to teach us cutting-edge information. I grab for the trinkets, the pens and pads of paper, and then, minutes later, I cannot remember what the drug is used for.

I used to think I needed to be out in the hall, listening to a doctor talk with all the other white coats about the importance of some test or the newest study. Now, it seems, I just answer call lights and take people off bedpans. I think sometimes this is why I am still here, after all. This thing I can do, I do well. I try to convey to a bedridden patient that the indignities our bodies create do not bother me and I will be there to help. Sometimes I tell them of my own hospital stay, of how I, too, was embarrassed to have my body and all its functions out for public view.

When I go home, I am at peace with myself. I'm not the smartest, fastest, certainly not the youngest nurse who works here. I can sleep best when I know that I was there when my patients needed me.

Very soon, I will go one last time to the parking lot. And it will be okay, even if only I know that I did this work well.

READING THE INSTRUCTIONS FIRST

It seems the most important things we do in life are left untaught, unexplained. We are told to refrain from sex, but not how to be a mom or dad. We are told how to breathe during contractions, "Hee, hee, hee, whew!" But not how to breathe when we get the call at 2:00 a.m. that our child has been picked up for drunk driving. We are told not to squander our money on electronic games when we are 13 years old, and how to solve for X in algebra, (something which I have never once actually needed to do in my adult life). But we grow up clueless about how to pay bills, save money, or negotiate a car loan or mortgage.

So it shouldn't be a surprise that we have no idea at all how to retire successfully. The leaders in this field are out of touch, in ill health or moved away. And, often, they do not talk about their success.

The job I have now is most likely my last. When I was young, I loved change and uncertainty. If one place didn't work out, I thought, "What luck!" I could go elsewhere. Interviewing well was all it took. My future seemed limited only by the number of copies I made of my resume.

The very thing I loved most in my twenties – being free, living away from family, having nothing to hold me back – now scares the hell out of me. My address book is filled with corrections, some entries lined out all together: death, divorce, disinterest.

If time marches on, it is stepping over fallen friends. Addresses changed, neighborhoods going downhill, sometimes an old place is quite literally plowed under for a new convenience store and parking lot. Gone. Remembered by only me, it would seem.

How to live in the present and not dwell on the past? How to keep looking forward without seeing the aura of what has gone before in our peripheral vision?

Volunteer work has its limits. If you were used to being in charge, having some control, pushing forward to make improvements, it is more difficult to swallow this new pill. The common denominator is larger, the mix diluted. Start times are suggestions, not a reason for dismissal. And many volunteer assignments seem to be a form of fundraising. Unless you were an entrepreneur before retiring, this can be a daunting task, making you feel like a small ant trying to carry the breadcrumb uphill. No matter how well-meant the organization is, it needs money to keep going, and it is to you they will turn to provide it.

The most vital people I have met in my work as a nurse were still working in their later life. Even much later. A 94-year old man still went to his son's dental practice every day to help make plaster molds for orthodontia. He had a place to go, every day. He had routine, and a reason to buy new clothes, to stop for a bag of donuts, and a secretary to honor with flowers each season. He was *not* talking about his own health each day. Or, only a very little.

A woman was the receptionist at the local Hospice office until late August. Then, her income would exceed the limit for her to receive her Social Security money. She really *ran* the office and she was happy to tell us later that it fell apart while she was gone each fall. Things were immaculate under her watch. But her toughness evaporated the minute she answered the phones. She knew what it meant to need to call the office for help, having lost her husband in our care.

Most of us can't work part-time quite so easily, I suppose. But all work is honorable and there are clearly many jobs to do in our community. What of tutoring children after school? What about respite care so a family member can have a break? Dog- or house-sitting? Or the care needed to open a cottage?

Still, it seems there should be a class available on how to age gracefully. Even without one, I suspect I will be okay. I assembled all my first years without reading the instructions; why would the rest be any different?

On a country road I travel frequently, I have seen a baby red-tailed hawk sitting on a road sign – fluffing his wings in the wind. He appears to be practicing. Maybe it will be like that for me. I'll learn to fly when I retire, by putting out my wings and letting go. Even if I can't read the sign.

LATE STAGES

As if they had some whispered announcement, "young people only," hospitals are staffed with youth. The work is not barrier-free. And it is not the hospital's call to provide a pasture for older nurses. So the aged leave and our staff has few who remember hospital stays counted in weeks and days instead of hours.

At 35, you begin to have doubts. As you get your coat on in the locker room you are reminded by the oncoming staff member that you have some charting to catch up on. Actually, for one patient, you have not put one word on paper. At 40, your bad days start in earnest. By now you are wearing glasses and shoe inserts and worry about forgetting something important all the time. At 45, there is growing frustration: the betrayal you feel toward a profession that cares for the sick and elderly and dying but does not hesitate to gnaw off its own foot when caught in a trap, the vice-like grip of the increasing workload. There were no promises that day long ago when you hired in; no one told you they would ease up on your work as you were able to do less and less.

Your co-workers are having babies and you're having hot flashes. You constantly find yourself walking to the desk or storage room or equipment holding area, and not being sure why you are there. Your mind is shot, your body slowing, your patients and their families are asking for more and more. At 55, you will be desperate to go – anywhere. Work you never thought of before will look better. Work that allows a chair now and then, a place that doesn't cause the adrenaline to run wide open in your veins. Maybe something with humane hours and some place that doesn't have 300-pound people that need to be helped off gurneys.

But now you have found even more reasons to stay. Your children have become expensive, maybe a son is in grad school or your daughter is planning a wedding reception for 400. And there won't be a nest egg of money on which to retire unless you have earned it for yourself. At 60, you simply will not be there anymore. Maybe you've gone to a physician's office, (not for your own illness!) or are taking histories for an insurance company. But gone from what you thought you would do forever when you started.

It's like the contract for an injured baseball player. If you are benched, you can't do bedside care. I tried asking my co-workers about this aging business. I polled them, asking, "If six nurses were assigned to the unit, would it be okay if two of them were over 50 and couldn't do quite as much as the 25-year olds?" I also gave a little speech about the need for experience, the balance and calming influence, the large body of knowledge older workers bring. The answers were: 1) No; 2) No; 3) I don't know; 4) Yah, sure, especially if I were one of the 50-year-olds; and 5) Hey, turn your head to the light. Do you know you have chin hair?

My husband helpfully offered that maybe our unit needed a greeter at the door, like Wal-

Mart. Or someone like the ladies at McDonald's who go around with coffee refills. These ideas were not well received.

Sometimes I think of the very, very few who have stayed and I admire them, not for their stamina, but for their skill. Every now and then, one lingers and does well. They stay but do not stagnate. They remain strong, but do not calcify.

Growing old is not for sissies. As a nurse, I have watched up close the dramatic reversals the human body makes. We are given youth and health and then, like a dripping candle, it slowly melts away. We won't get out of this alive. Our bodies are supposed to change. And it is not sad to find that we have had our chance at being young and now, that chance is someone else's.

The problem for each of us is how to leave gracefully. To have said our lines and done our part and stepped down off the stage without making an ugly scene. To walk away from nursing and be missed and remembered fondly.

It is tempting to point out what is wrong. How someone younger is not as respectful, or lacks skills. It is easy to get used to benefits and higher wages as one progresses in the system. And to believe that somehow the organization owes me a softer job. After all the years I have given them. But, while positions do become available elsewhere in the hospital, bedside nursing is just that: meeting the needs of the acutely ill, bedridden patient. This isn't changing any time soon, not even for one staff member because her feet hurt or her shoulder is strained. Just as it is not the hospital's fault that you live an hour away and must occasionally come in on your day off for in-services. The hospital is not a friendly uncle who can fix everything for the whole family. There is a reason they call it work. And, in our case, hard work.

The job now is to find something to take the place of what I have loved doing for so long. Something as satisfying as being someone's nurse. To have helped people with the transitions in their lives, to have worked with wonderful co-workers who always pitched in, to have gotten up each morning and looked forward to the day, to have been available for family while working around my small children's lives, and to know when I put my head down each night on the pillow that I have been kind and smart and caring and gentle and my work has made a difference.

This will be such a hard act to follow. But I count myself lucky to have ever found this wonderful work at all.

OLD POOP!

Getting older is like when the toilet paper roll is getting low and each sheet doesn't seem to count for much. And actually, you can't even see the difference in just one sitting. But after a while, it's not your imagination, it IS getting low. And you know that, someday, you're going to use that last sheet and probably you'll still have more to do.

THINGS YOU WILL NEVER KNOW

So much of nursing is invisible. Or almost, it would seem. We are there at your beginning and end, and witness to so much of what goes on in between.

Some years ago, my younger son fell asleep driving home in the early morning hours. According to the man that witnessed the scene and stopped, my son rolled his car seven times. The entire passenger compartment was crushed; there could not have been room for my 6'2" son, my big red-headed man-child. But he walked away, with only one scratch to his elbow. I still cannot tell you why we were not picking out a coffin that same day. It was a kind of miracle – a set of circumstances put in place by people who had gone before and made it possible for my son to live.

I wanted to look up the names of the inventors of the seatbelt and the shoulder harness, and the road engineers who knew to carve the shoulder with a gentle berm. I thought about going back in time to the 1950s and seeing some thoughtful scientist in his geeky black-rimmed glasses and pocket protector with pencils sticking out, and I would rush up to him and hug him, and we both would be embarrassed. My son survived because of him. I was grateful for the invisible people who made this possible.

I too do work that is invisible. I am paid by the hour by my hospital, a part of the "hotel costs."

And each day I work, I never know for whom I will care. But as a nurse, like all the nurses I work with, I feel that I am called to do battle with each patient's disease. Without judgment. With kindness. To genuinely care.

So many things a nurse does are things you will never know. To check your labs, call a doctor, adjust an IV. To give you medications or not to give them when we know it would be wrong. To turn and position and comfort you. To give you dignity even in the most undignified moments.

It is likely that a nurse first cleaned the birthing fluids from your little face, moments after you were born. It could easily be a nurse that will wipe your brow or hold your hand when you take your last breath. I have been making coffee with a patient's wife as we talked about hair color, and then minutes later, I have called a code and found myself doing compressions on the lifeless chest of her husband. I have taught about disease and shown movies and given pamphlets. But then, at discharge, I see my patient on the way to his car, lighting up a cigarette, and know I will see him again, soon.

We will be here. We, as a group, never have a day off. The care you will receive, the day you need a nurse will, quite literally, be the best there is. That nurse, that day, will give you all she has. Cumulatively, we are the outcome of research and trial and error, centuries of learning and finding best outcomes. And much of your care will be invisible.

Though our profession has many advanced-practice levels with long educational paths and great accomplishments, the nurse you will most likely meet will be the one at your bedside, in a hospital. He or she will be your friend and confidante, the eyes and ears for the doctor who sees you only briefly and then moves on, and the cheerleader as you progress to get well.

Sometimes when I go to a party with my husband and there are no nurses there, I know I won't be able to talk about my work. It's complicated and so real: life and death are the bottom line, not profit and loss. By being personal, so much so, that even priests do not hear what I am told. By being broken-hearted from the pain I sometimes witness, and knowing that no narcotic will help. By being called to be a silent witness to a life, and help in quiet ways that matter but that do not show.

Many times, you will not remember our names or know that we were there. You will tell your friends of the great surgeon who straightened out your crooked leg, or the doctor who got you started on the medication that finally worked and you will go home from the hospital with your health improved.

If the scientists that made a nylon belt and grassy knoll to keep my son alive were invisible, why shouldn't I be? I am honored to be a part of every patient's story, to be a witness as someone's life unfolds. And to be a part of the things they do not know.

Katie MacInnis is a registered nurse at Northern Michigan Hospital in Petoskey, Michigan. She works on a cardiovascular floor, but has worked in OB-Peds, Hospice, homecare, and ICU in the years since 1981 when she received her degree from Lansing Community College. Prior to this, she received a BA from Alma College in English and art. She and her husband Charlie live in Harbor Springs and have two grown sons, Scott and Rob.

Katie's stories have been published in RN Excellence and the American Journal of Nursing. Over the years, her friends have told her that they have found Xeroxed copies of her stories in their orientation syllabus at new hospitals, in the ancillary reading for a death and dying class at a state university and as part of the curriculum for a nursing school class.

It is great to be published, but an honor to be Xeroxed!

Feel free to contact Katie at:
8440 Blackberry Trail
Harbor Springs, Michigan 49740.
Phone 231-526-1557
e-mail: katiemac@core.com